ABOUT THE AUTHOR

Paula Burns is a Midlands' based artist and writer. Before taking early retirement, due to a neurological condition, she worked as a psychotherapist and was engaged in research studies in the Philosophy Department at the University of Warwick. Her first novel 'Blue-Grey Island' (an exploration of dementia) was published by Matador in 2012. Paula's art work and poetry can be viewed at her website www.paulaburns.co.uk

CONVERSATIONS WITH LEOPARD

PAULA BURNS

Matador
9 Priory Business Park,
Wistow Road, Kibworth Beauchamp,
Leicestershire. LE8 0RX
Tel: (+44) 116 279 2299
Fax: (+44) 116 279 2277
Email: books@troubador.co.uk
Web: www.troubador.co.uk/matador

ISBN 978 1783065 400

British Library Cataloguing in Publication Data.
A catalogue record for this book is available from the British Library.

Typeset in 11pt Aldine401 BT Roman by Troubador Publishing Ltd, Leicester, UK

Matador is an imprint of Troubador Publishing Ltd

This story is rooted in memoir and magic realism. The narrative is an imaginative re-creation of events in my life and a re-telling of family history that has been passed down in the form of stories, letters and diaries.

There is no intention to portray events in a factual or chronological order or present an accurate portrayal of any individual – living or deceased.

Some names have been changed.

For Simon and Emma

&

Lana and Owen,
who believe in the magic of stories
the existence of Tinkerbell
and Leopards who talk.

'A memoir is how one remembers one's life …'

Gore Vidal, 'Palimpsest – A Memoir –'

'The ordinariness of magic realism's magic relies on its accepted and unquestioned position in tangible and material reality.'

Maggie Ann Bowers, 'Magic(al) Realism
(The New Critical Idiom)'

'I've built a grass hut where there's nothing of value.
After eating, I relax and enjoy a nap.
When the hut was completed, fresh weeds appeared.
Now it's been lived in-covered with weeds.
The person in the hut lives here calmly,
not stuck to inside, outside, or in-between.
Places worldly people live, he doesn't live.
Realms worldly people love, she doesn't love.
Though the hut is small, it includes the whole world.'

'Song of the Grass-Roof Hermitage' by Shitou Xiqian (700-790)★

★*From 'Cultivating the Empty Field' by Taigen Dan Leighton.*

(Permission to quote granted by Tuttle Publishing).

No other truth but my own is conveyed by this story.

A Vignette from Childhood
1963

I picture myself as a child – a girl of eleven years of age.

The child is stood facing a wall – alongside a small group of fellow pupils. The children pose – fixed and silent – as they wait excitedly for the unveiling of a portrait of the Queen. The young girl tightly clutches a piece of paper from which she has just read a presentation speech to the mayor.

I cannot remember the content of the speech but at some point the word *proud* must have been uttered.

The child feels a sense of pride in being chosen to read her own words to the assembled council dignitaries – but the acquisition of a new pair of shoes plays uppermost.

I have a recollection of pleading with my mother to buy the cherry-red sandals instead of the usual boring, brown brogues. It was quite a triumph when she finally gave in.

The youngster wriggles her toes, whilst surreptitiously

admiring a pretty daisy pattern of tiny dots punched into the red patent leather. Waiting for the auspicious moment of the unveiling is fidget provoking. The head teacher – smartly attired and well groomed – steps forward, and deftly pulls the red tassel at the side of a small curtain. The child thinks of a similar curtain on a Punch and Judy theatre she'd seen at the sea-side, during an annual holiday. A biting north wind had ripped through her thin summer dress that day. But her father enthusiastically inhaled the cold air and murmured something about his beloved Tyneside – exiled as they were the rest of the year in a warmer Midlands' clime.

The plush velvet screen parts to reveal an oil painting of Her Majesty – who seems to direct her gaze towards the audience with a beneficent smile.

I remember a boy positioned in front of me. Classmates and friends, since the age of four, the boy and I might once have huddled in close proximity. Our respective names – Paula and Paul – are an easy combination of sounds that naturally trip off the tongue. But recently we have been teased. The pop song *Hey Paula* is top of the hit parade and for weeks the other children have giggled and pointed at us, crooning the lyrics at every opportunity.

Sometimes childhood sucks!

The local journalists scribe with their pens and a photographer illuminates the room with blue, luminescent flashes of light. It is, in fact, all over in a flash.

My mother saved the newspaper clipping and a copy of the photograph, for she was no doubt proud. But all that can be seen is the back of my head, held at a certain tilt, as I gaze up at the portrait.

The child is aware her time at Primary school is almost over and of a worrying correlation between this encroaching event and an ominous sense that the *magic* is fading. Lying in bed – in the darkness – she still sees the floating bubbles of light, a strange phenomenon that had mysteriously appeared to her at the age of four. The bubbles are the colours of the rainbow and shine with neon brightness as they float and dart around the bedroom with dizzying speed. But her other magical powers are clearly diminishing. She can no longer bring her dolls and teddies to life and the fairy called Tinker Bell – who she once willed into her dreams from the pages of Peter Pan – has vanished. The child's imagination disappears down a black hole of nightmares, fuelled by the pressure of being schooled to pass tests concocted from the horrors of mental arithmetic and problem solving.

One night, in deep sleep – just as she has given up on magic – the child discovers flight, an exhilarating sensation as her body lifts effortlessly from the bed. Higher she soars through the earth's heavy atmosphere, suddenly gaining speed as her senses enter a space of ultimate weightlessness and intense light.

Years pass by and the child gradually forgets how to fly. The floating bubbles of light also fade into the grey nothingness of a monochrome night-time backdrop. Then one morning, after hours of fitful dreams, she wakes with the realisation that her childhood has been swallowed up by the passage of time and how her adult self is trapped within a carapace as dull as the rejected brown brogues. The second skin pinches – tight and brittle – and she decides to search for the lost, playful child.

This is the point where my story begins, a place where the past merges with the present and the present is always slipping away.

PART ONE

(1990-2000)

ONE

The Leopard's Desire

I am removed. Is anyone apart from Matthew aware of this fact? Or do people say, 'We saw her just the other day – she seems to be coping.'

I cope therefore I am.

In the secret spaces of my mind that allow for the gut reaction to pain, the verb *to cope* is abolished. There is a strange creature with long tentacles residing in my brain. The tentacles sliver and squeeze tightening their grip around my forehead. Phrases like *sensory overload* take on a startling clarity.

In truth – there is little clarity these days as words slip and stumble. I ask Matthew for a trowel 'with holes'. He smiles at my latest word confusion and hands me a garden fork. I give a little laugh but inwardly I'm sighing. I have no idea what I'm going to do with the garden implement but it makes me feel better holding an object that at least indicates *the intention* of purpose – while Matthew gets on with the genuine task of planting spring flowers. Where is the articulate and energetic woman he married less than a year ago?

My children are also bemused. Right now, I'm satisfied if I can manage to get dressed and produce a tray of flapjacks for afternoon tea. This is not the multi-tasking mother they're used to, though I'm aiming for some degree of normality – seeking comfort in the domestic routine we shared when they were little. But two teenagers, well used to their independence and personal space, possibly don't require this overt attention to my trying to be there for them.

As for Matthew, he must feel like he co-exists in some far-away-place – quite removed from the life we'd anticipated. As newlyweds, we made our vows just eight months ago and found ourselves immediately put to the test.

Friends who attended the happy occasion are a little wide of the mark and observe in passing, 'Matthew's Ok – though he's very busy working away from home. Still – he seems cheery enough.'

I work therefore I am.

This is the creed of the twentieth century as our planet hurtles towards the new millennium. A more comforting rendition of existence will hardly suffice, for spirit has long been removed from the equation. Reason remains, detached from the comforting presence of spirit. To work and to cope, this is the definition of existence.

It is difficult to express the loneliness not existing entails. This troubling thought chatters away in my head during our weekly shopping trip as I pick my way through cans of baked beans. I smile, directing my gaze beyond curious stares and attempt to appear *normal.* The sense of guilt attached to not getting better often proves disorientating.

The beans clatter into the shopping trolley, startling me and causing my lips to instinctively curl. I have to be careful not to snarl! My human form is momentarily enveloped within the body of a leopard – a male leopard. This invisible metamorphosis is becoming a regular occurrence and the change of gender is strangely pleasing.

I experience a sense of empowerment as shaking arms reach down within the sinewy outline of the creature's front legs and trembling fingers stretch to make contact with soft padded paws. An aching spine elongates and relaxes in response to the sensation of a silky fur coat replacing tight human skin. Then, as if by a miracle, previously weakened legs purposively push down into the leopard's hindquarters. Saliva fills my mouth, accompanied by the increasing urge to snarl and lash out with a powerful paw. And all of this time a pair of yellow-green eyes carefully watch whilst my leopard brain buzzes with the instinct of caution and the desire for stealth. The desire of the leopard is focused on stealth for without stealth there is death.

I feel scarcely human these days.

Sometimes the leopard feels wholly part of me and at other times he's just *out there* – occupying his own physical space. It's true this space is circumscribed because the creature is unable to move further than the distance I can gauge with my human eye. I like to think that one day my confined companion will break free and become completely autonomous; so it's only fair to speak of him as Leopard with a capital L, a fully-fledged being in his own right.

When I'm with Leopard the natural environment takes on a different slant. There is nothing forced or alienating in this – it's more like a whisper you've been struggling to decipher becoming a clear voice. The cosmos is full of whispering. For example, the sun takes on her innate disposition when Leopard is there to hear her speak. In Leopard's world to call Sun *'the sun'* is highly disrespectful and so it is with Moon.

At home, in the garden, Sun is hiding behind the fir trees. In my child's mind, which is also my spirit mind, I dress up in a net-layered skirt – crinkly and twinkling with the sparkle of sequins and skip and twirl. There is no guilt attached to doing nothing, achieving nothing of particular intent. The spirit child stares at my adult self quizzically and asks, 'What is *nothing?*'

Leopard searches for this playful state of nothingness as he paces back and forth in a cage, frustrated with his incapacity to circle three hundred and sixty degrees with Sun. So much dappling of leaves and glistening of water is being missed. And what of the movement of air – discernible within the bending, twisting and rustling of branches, leaves and grasses? What of the caress of a warm breeze – or the harsh bite of a winter chill on exposed skin? Leopard misses it all yet his whole being contracts from this amazing perceptual world of sight, sound, touch, taste and smell.

Sun shimmers through the dense foliage of the fir trees. Leopard sighs as the object of his desire gradually disappears behind the slanted rooftops. The creature waits with the tenacity of a lover, knowing this caprice is part of what it must endure.

'*So Leopard's real object of desire is an uninterrupted view of Sun?*'

'*Yes – that and the capacity for stealth. Stealth is the desire of Leopard focused inwards.*'

TWO

1992
Celestial Sisters

It is the creature's second autumn trapped within the cage. Sun has been particularly flirtatious the past year, warming Leopard's soft coat until late October and still making an appearance during the normally bleak month of November.

Sun has a rival, a competitor who shadows her every move in an effort to ensnare Leopard's affections. The creature's response is not based upon reason, for he took time to realise that the globe, which hung mysteriously in the sky at night, was not Sun attired in a beguiling dress of pale yellow.

Leopard sniffs the cool night air and feels a sensation deep in his instinctual soul. Like a far distant cry, which is barely audible, the sound of rushing water cascades within his ears. A fraction of a second later sound joins with visual movement to become an image. The creature sees itself running; running swiftly along a riverbank accompanied by Moon's luminous light.

Leopard once heard it muted that Sun and Moon are either jealous sisters, or an estranged mother and daughter. Sun and Moon stick to the sister genealogy, though Moon is often disquieted by the opposing rumour.

Sun couldn't care less; being the eldest she has always taken advantage of her superiority. Sun boasts of being destined to give warmth and light to a segment of time known by humans as *day,* whilst timid, inferior Moon is allotted the task of illuminating the darkness known as *night.*

Moon rails against her fate – arguing night is too quiet a space for her to inhabit. She reasons her sister will always bask in the admiration of the humans who love to loll around semi-naked, just waiting for Sun to shine upon them.

It took Moon many centuries to create an aura of mystery. Her constant lament is her failure to realise, at the dawn of her creation, the power of her luminosity.

Sun's attitude hasn't exactly helped her sister's lack of self-esteem.

'Hah!' she remarks, in a smug tone of voice Moon recognises only too well. 'The humans know you don't have your own light – that all you do is to reflect mine. If it wasn't for me you'd be completely in the dark!'

Moon's anger depleted her spirit and she languished in fear, sensing an age was to come when humankind would walk upon the contours of her body only to discover these were nothing more than dry bones and ashes. Also, try as she might to ignore rumour, the interplanetary gossip niggles. She once heard it insinuated that Sun is really the mother of Earth and her poor self is the rejected offspring of Earth.

'That would make me your grandmother,' Sun smirks, with some relish.

'Well, sometimes …' Moon winces, 'the human's talk of a daughter as being like a sister – but I haven't heard it said that a grandmother may feel as though a granddaughter is a sister.'

'Oh – what the heck!' Sun shrugs. 'We're stuck with each other – so sisters it is.'

The sisters keep their distance and it is only at certain times, in a space designated *early evening*, the tension between them may be visualised. Sun bleeds into evening whilst Moon adopts a series of images. Sometimes she poses as a cuticle of pale coloured tissue paper and at others a semicircle of deeper hue. Her true sensuality is only evident at the time of *full moon*, an event during which Moon's rage at her lost potency sends shock waves which are intuited by certain sensitive humans.

Leopard remembers an image of freedom, an image possessing such clarity he has difficulty in thinking of it as truly located within the past. Within Leopard's brain I understand how the notion of time may slip through its own boundaries – that the interrelationship between time and space can be mysteriously prized apart.

My companion positions himself in front of the ticking clock – head rested on outstretched paws. He sits for a long time, pensively observing the second hand's circular trajectory. Then he focuses attention on the minute hand as it jolts from stationary to sudden movement – like an annoying fly's erratic take off on sensing the imminent whack of a fly swatter.

'You can't swat a minute without observing the second hand,' he muses, 'and as for the hour – not possible without observing the minutes. That's if you need to be exact.'

'Can you swat a minute merely by stealth?'

'Maybe – think of it as like stalking a gazelle – or any object of prey. If you observe with patience it becomes evident when to pounce.'

'But,' I ask – puzzled, 'what would be the purpose of capturing time?'

'No purpose at all, except humans are peculiar – dividing their lives into smaller and smaller segments, all defined by time. They like to put all the little segments into boxes and then store them in some dusty attic called the mind.'

'Well time does have its uses Leopard – humans can't live in the real world without a notion of time … and it would be odd not to have memories.'

Leopard scratches his nose and rolls over. 'What's the *real* world? In the jungle I was free – I hunted when hungry and slept when tired. Nature's time is different to human time.'

'I get what you mean Leopard – and given my situation it doesn't exactly help to quantify my life's experiences through the passage of time.'

Leopard stretches and licks a paw in readiness for his morning grooming session. 'Ok – what happens if you try to figure your life purely in terms of space?'

I think on this before rushing to reply. 'Well … I would have to say I exist within a strange, bewildering space – a timeless space – because although I can mark its beginning, in the way we might mark the event of a human conception, I have no way of marking an end – other than by death. And even death's not a certainty because I do not fully understand what death as an experience entails.'

Leopard yawns and settles down on his favourite blanket.

He accepts having started this conversation he's in for the long haul – especially as the twin spectres of mortality and the passage of time have been introduced!

'Beginnings and endings – a tricky subject,' he concedes. 'Do you have anything else to add before I have a nap?'

'Only that I long to escape time – because the notion of time haunts me more than this illness. When people say, 'this will pass,' what do they mean? Do they mean this time will pass or this space will pass? I am always in this space, time passes but the space does not.'

Leopard is looking a bit sleepy but I try to hold his attention.

'When I was a child I had a favourite book entitled *When the Clock Stood Still.*'

This perks him up as he likes stories. 'Go on then,' he encourages.

'In the story, a clock in a children's nursery stops marking time at the stroke of midnight. The children enter a magical world where the toys in the nursery come alive. Eradicating time protects their playful space.'

'Mmmm … and the connection?'

'This is the kind of perimeter placed around me by illness. I no longer inhabit the same space as humans who live within the boundaries of a strong connection between space and time. To talk about my life in terms of past, present and future seems flimsy, inadequate.'

Leopard sits erect for a few seconds – with one paw held in mid-air. He is thinking.

'In that case,' he tentatively suggests, whilst finishing washing with a quick polish of his whiskers, 'it's of little consequence if we sleep all through the day though the rest of the world is busy?'

'I guess not,' I sigh, curling up beside him, 'but …' I whisper, close to his ear, 'there was a beginning – a time when I became you and you became me.'

THREE

Leopards Don't Travel On The Tube

Once upon a time I worked as a psychotherapist.

My career gave me a passport to an existence in the material world – a world pulsating with new opportunities and challenges.

I am nostalgic for the pleasures of freedom and success from within the present limitations of the cage. Yet Leopard's mind will not allow me to stay stuck with this thought. Leopard's mind has contrary memories which break into my state of reverie.

'What is it that you miss?' Leopard enquires, though he's fully cognisant of the impending inventory.

'I miss not being able to walk: to drive my car distances: to stay awake for more than a few hours at a time: to socialise with friends, family and colleagues: to be mentally stimulated by my work and – most of all – I miss the sense of being needed and valued.'

Leopard gazes out of the window at the autumn sunlight dappling the remaining leaves on semi-clad trees. He gazes for a long time pondering on the gaps in my account of loss.

He knows I do not lie, that the loss is genuine. But he also forces me to acknowledge how the desire for stealth was germinating within my thoughts and perceptions, like a grain of mustard seed, before I became obviously sick.

'Do you remember,' he probes, 'the exact moment when you began to turn into me?'

'Absolutely,' I reply, as we continue to imprint the image of autumn sunshine in readiness for our winter sojourn.

It all began one day as I travelled to London by train. Having bought my ticket, and a magazine to read in the waiting room, the usual routine was to people watch over a polystyrene cup of British Rail tea. This activity was not particularly voyeuristic – but more to do with a genuine enjoyment in observing the little idiosyncrasies of my fellow commuters. I struggled to people watch that day due to an unnerving sense that I had become the sole object of *their* observation, and that by some mysterious process my external body had suffered an erasure of any defining marks of being human.

Despite an autumn chill the poorly heated waiting room suddenly transformed into a furnace. The woollen jacket, chosen for warmth, now felt as though it was lined with pine needles pricking and irritating my sweating skin. Worse still, a flapping sensation over my heart convinced me a small bird must be trapped within the layers of clothing and was desperately trying to escape. A whiff of the scent of human bodies assailed my nostrils and my stomach churned in response to the troupe of dancing butterflies, fluttering, twisting and swirling within its empty, cavernous space.

A voice boomed over the tannoy system at the precise moment air-starved lungs – belonging to whatever creature I had become – contracted with panic in response to a desire to escape – to escape from what? *Danger!* … my body registered danger as I fled the waiting room and paced up and down the platform seeking solid ground. The sound of the approaching train magnified and the sight of the engine and carriages was transposed into a vision of an ominous spectral object, moving closer and closer until it finally hurtled and screeched towards a halt. I stood terrorised at the edge of the platform.

How to regain composure despite the inner conviction that something or someone was out to capture me? This animal instinct grew stronger as I cautiously surveyed the other passengers boarding the train. Sinking down into my seat I inwardly debated who the predator might be? Was it the slimy looking businessman now sat opposite, with his polished shoes and sickening smell of aftershave? Or maybe the tousled young man hugging his holdall and listening to a Walkman – but watching, stalking me out of the corner of his eye?

I eluded capture but later that day the tube journey proved even more perilous. Hyper-sensitized skin instinctively tightened in response to the forced body contact with all those humans. This was the start of many nightmare journeys to and from London. In the space between I sat in a small, cosy therapy room and saw clients. Inside, I felt distinctly ill at ease. An intense desire for physical movement – to sing and dance – continually threatened to break an imposed still and silent position. My arms felt heavy with the weight of holding an imaginary baby close to my heart, for there was a symbiotic relationship of need between this infant and myself.

Who could have predicted that like the baby in Alice in Wonderland, which strangely morphed into a pig, this baby was to change into a leopard – a leopard destined to be caged? No one – except perhaps a shaman? A shaman may have seen the net slowly flung and cautioned how the sick, empty sensation in the pit of the stomach was an instinctive, primal warning of impending capture. There is a dearth of shamans in North London and I *was* caught.

It would be unfair to say that others had not tried to intervene. A user-friendly doctor kindly made a relaxation tape and delivered it by hand. My human self is still touched by this but Leopard could not relate to the mellifluous voice, the imperative to relax within the calm ambience of a beautiful garden. All that sniffing of herbaceous borders and attuning of the ears to sweet little fountains!

Leopard's whiskers twitched in disdain! Where was the jungle, the lush vegetation, the shrieking of parakeets and cascading of waterfalls?

Too late … Leopard fails to find his way home. During the winter of 1989, London is situated at the epicentre of the viral pool. With insidious intent a microscopic spore enters Leopard's nostrils. He sneezes, he coughs, he gently paws his moist eyes. The limbs are heavy, they ache, refuse to move. Sinew and bone seize up.

The virus was only meant to last a couple of weeks – a minuscule particle in the structure of time given to me as my life. The particle broke free; it broke free from time and took my life with it. Days, weeks, months, years … none of these terms for marking the events of my life apply anymore.

It doesn't really matter it is the second year in the cage.
It is simply autumn once again.

FOUR

1993
Moon's Exotic Dance

Seasons pass – clouds drift by…

Sun dances high in the sky, her warm rays glistening through the conservatory roof and casting a luminous glow on the leaves of the plants. The soft greens vie for attention against the blood red impatiens. Matthew and I have brought part of the garden inside before the winter frosts bite.

The conservatory is an important aspect of my sanctuary having yielded its hoards of books and notes. One by one the folders were pushed further towards the edge of the large pine desk.

'No room!' the trays of seedlings cried, 'what need has paper and words for Sun's warmth?'

Each morning my eyes are drawn to the hibiscus plant. This hibiscus is extraordinary because it strives to unfold one purple bloom at a time. I have grown to love such singularity of purpose.

Purple fails to describe the colour of a hibiscus bloom. Purple is just an inefficient word. As years pass, words begin to crumble into ambivalent units of sound – sounds which slip through Leopard's mind. *Friend* becomes *fiend* – *kiss* becomes *cuss*. Leopard lives through his senses. Pictures in the space between his yellow-green eyes help him to survive.

DARK DAY FOR RATIONALISTS AS ECLIPSE CROSSES ASIA
The Guardian – Oct. 1993

The external world has slithered under the door in the guise of the newspaper. I keep on with reading about this material realm – a realm I no longer feel fully part of. There is something 'out there' I still care about but what, I ask myself, has happened to its connection with me?

Leopard is getting twitchy; soon he will be snarling that it's no use having this internal dialogue because I will only lapse into self-pity.

Self-pity is the raw underbelly of loneliness. Self-pity is the whimper in the dark that is a cry for help.

Leopard stalks up and down, as he does when trying to remind me of stealth – how it is dangerous to wander too long in the company of such thoughts.

I turn my mind to the antics of Sun and Moon. Moon is in raptures over the reviews of her performance. The tabloids are full of how she had 'danced' across Sun just after dawn. She remembers the location – the first act had begun in central Iran where she took centre stage in the sky. A graceful opening movement progressed to an exotic, speedy dance over Burma. Moon loved the sense of exhilaration and choreographed the next part of the spectacle to include a lively gavotte across Vietnam, northern Malaysia and Indonesia – during which she grabbed the odd unsuspecting cloud or sleeping star to partner her. The power of it!

Moon is elated at her sudden surge of self-esteem but Sun is most put out. How to bear the shame? Sun doesn't relish the rationalist explanations giving full credence to her sister. She longs for the continuation of an ancient mythology that 'swears to the demon which flies across her surface and plunges the eastern hemisphere into darkness'.

FIVE

1994
The Magic Chocolate Tree

Time passes. Leopard observes yet another autumn give way to winter as his coat thickens against the biting wind. A few remaining leaves are snatched from the trees, like bodies stripped of any vestiges of personal signification. The oak: the apple: the orange blossom – all laid bare – their branches reaching out like skeletal arms and hands with fingers devoid of jewelled finery.

The creature shivers as snow clouds darken the sky. It is the prelude to the winter dance of Sun and Moon, each competing to produce a scene of snowy splendour. The garden sparkles with frosted whiteness throwing a canopy over Leopard's brain. Leopard sees the image of a little girl projected onto the canopy – a soft-edged image lacking the sharpness of a material human form.

The child jumps up and down in the snow, freeing her hands from mittens which are loosely threaded through the sleeves of her coat.

'Who puts the sparkly bits in the snow?' she enquires of a man, slipping icy fingers into the palm of his warm hand.

'The snow fairies.'

The child giggles, covering her mouth in astonishment.

'Daddy,' she demands, bolder now, 'how, how do they do that?'

'Whenever the fairies fly across the sky their wings shed a thousand drops of silvery particles that fall to the ground below.'

The man reaches for a handful of powdery snow and throws it up into the air. 'Like this,' he cries.

'But why can't we see the fairies?' the little girl persists, copying her father's gesture.

'It wouldn't be magic if we could see them – would it?' he smiles.

Only half-satisfied with this answer the child marches, struggling to keep cold, damp feet in a pair of over-sized, squelchy wellies that are a hand-me-down from her big sister. Two pigtails emerge from the rim of a woolly hat and fall down her back.

'Daddy, shall we have hot Bovril when we get home?'

'Indeed we will,' her father replies, rubbing his hands together and laughing, 'indeed we will.'

But first they must continue with their adventure; Leopard knows this. In the space between his yellow-green eyes he sees a pond frozen over and his ears are sensitive to the acoustics of pebble and stone on fractured ice. The child presses the edge of the ice with her welly. She dreams of a pair of ice skates and a white, flowing dress adorned with swan feathers. Within this magical, wintry world, she is a swan skimming the surface of the ice with natural grace.

A second later the daydream is broken by the recollection of the promise given to her sister to make a snowman in the garden; and then she thinks of her mother waiting with fresh woollen socks, hung out to warm on the fireguard which is placed in front of a welcoming coal fire stoked up in the sitting room at home.

Leopard sighs. What can he do to keep the child in his garden – this garden that has become the sum totality of the external world? And yet the garden is never really the concrete world; it is a shimmering, ethereal landscape lit by Sun during the shortened winter days and illuminated by Moon on frosted winter nights.

There are many occasions when Sun and Moon do not oblige, days when Sun refuses to get her act together and nights when Moon sulks behind a black, silk screen. Leopard flicks a switch with his heavy paw and man-made light illuminates the nudity of the orange blossom, in contrast to the copiously clothed fir trees.

Sun sniggers. 'Why bother at all?' she shrieks, so Moon can hear. 'Why bother at all if these humans create their own light?'

Leopard understands the caprice of Sun and Moon, which is a reaction to their love/hate relationship with humans. He beckons the child back into the space and to my delight she is carrying a bag of chocolate money. The coins are wrapped in silver and gold foil. The little girl carefully ties the coins, one by one, to the branches of the orange blossom. The gold foil sparkles and twinkles as the coins spin in the wind.

'They are like baby sun and moons,' the child smiles at us, and then – with a flick of her pigtails – is gone.

SIX

1995
The Croaking Of Frogs

Sometimes the winter sleep is heavy and long. The flimsy rush blind has been replaced by green velour, a dense curtain drawn between the bedroom window and a grey November sky.

A pounding headache and permanent sore throat censors the act of speaking. Limbs ache and burn beneath the duvet cover and I curl up tight, trying not to dwell on the obligation of being human, on the pressure of human relationships. The desire to sleep is overwhelming, to drift into unconsciousness as the rain changes from sleet to snow. I feel tiny and diminished like a small creature. I am a field mouse basking in the sunshine, swaying on a hammock of golden wheat. My mind longs to linger within the sleepy creature's prelude to hibernation.

Hibernation feels like dreaming – an ethereal dream which drifts into a peaceful space as the external world slips away. At times it feels easier to stay within this liminal state.

Leopard lifts his head and stares – a stare that does not lack compassion but nevertheless calls for a review of the situation.

'You can't stay in a liminal state,' he sighs, 'there is still so much to care about.'

Leopard often makes me cry at this point – but the tears are an appreciation for all I continue to value rather than a sense of loss. There still seems to be an immense gap between losing a lot and losing everything. Myriad threads continue to connect me to life and as the obvious threads are cut away the clearer the remaining structure becomes. This revelation is dazzling in its simplicity and clarity.

The creature has taught me to be angry; to hiss, snarl, protest and then to let the anger go. Feelings of despair pass – just as winter passes. I open the curtains and once again the garden is coming to life. The still air reverberates with a strange sound and on listening closely I realise the mysterious noise is the croaking of frogs.

Spring has arrived.

SEVEN

Pond Weed

Mounting my trusty blue steed I set off at a pace down the garden. There is a whirring and jarring as the stabilisers catch on the bumps in the lawn. The lawn is a patch of sweet meadow grass strewn with daisies, dandelions, buttercups and clover. I recollect cutting and raking the blades of grass in bare feet, each strand dried to straw in the summer's heat. Such energy in limbs that moved at will.

Prior to acquiring a mobility buggy, sadness over my garden ran deep. The inability to dig, weed and hoe evoked such a longing for the smell of newly turned earth! Seasons changed and I missed the blue-purple splash of bluebells in the part of the garden that must once have been open fields or an orchard. One hundred and fifty steps lay between my bed and heaven.

It is years later as I write this, but it feels strange to think in terms of years. Pick a dandelion and blow the soft floss. One, two, three, four, five – five puffs of air – that's how quickly the years pass. Five puffs of air later, on buying a battery-powered scooter, the distance between heaven and my bed ceased to exist.

Gradually, I gave up on control. The relationship with my garden had not been taken, only the ability to do everything in a particular way. In letting go I learnt about the uncertainty that hovers beneath the drive towards omnipotence. Not worrying about the dross released me to think more about design.

Perceived through Leopard's yellow-green eyes the landscape became a canvas to paint upon. The colours grew from tiny seeds and I was free to watch each plant evolve as my sense of time imperceptively slowed down. Anxiety over lack of mobility became replaced by a sense of wonder at being placed within a slow-motion film – where every movement is captured in its essence.

Holding a clenched fist before Leopard's face I gradually uncurl each finger, like the graceful unfolding of a fern – frond by frond. Together we acknowledge a miracle of nature.

The scooter transports us away from the confined bedroom space into the freedom of the garden. Following the sound of the frogs croaking takes us on a route past the lawn and the herbaceous borders. The pond is beyond the greenhouse, just past the fir trees over which Sun dances. It is positioned in front of a summerhouse which nestles in the shade of an old apple tree. Our whole world is less than a third of an acre.

Several spring seasons have passed since Leopard and I were first startled by the sound of croaking frogs, but the memory of that occasion (which happened to coincide with one of Sun's bad moods) remains clear.

27

Leopard dipped his paw into the chilly pond that had not yet warmed because Sun had been in a tantrum. She was still in a bad mood, 'extremely miffed' (as she complained to Moon) at the expectations of humans who always presented her with such tight schedules. The sulk continued over a particularly bad experience she'd endured at Lee Cove, in Devon. Not satisfied with Sun gracing the moor and valley with spectacular light the humans expected her to provide the backdrop to a car advert.

'Hah!' she'd hissed at Moon, 'all those cameramen with their additions of man-made light and an automobile. It's such a hideous symbol of twentieth century consumerism and love of engineered speed!'

'You should worry,' Moon complained, as night drew in and she began to take centre stage, 'tonight is a lunar eclipse. They're all gathered in the valley, watching and waiting for the moment when Earth comes between me and thee.'

Sun had a brief moment of sisterly concern but her thoughts soon returned to the vexed question of body image. Dithering over which dress to wear, she opted for the paler hue well into May. That spring day, when I first heard the frogs croaking, she had tired of such coyness having decided to sparkle on the water.

Leopard pawed at the pondweed, drawing a piece from the still surface of the water and holding it up to the light. The weed presented a lattice work of shimmering green; an intricate woven structure of crisscrossing strands from which hung a delicate transparent matting formed from lime-green algae. Leopard and I were transfixed by this image, as we have been every following spring. A newt popped its head out of the latticework and then slivered upon the surface before plopping back into the pond.

The pondweed finds a way into my dreams. It has become a long piece of fabric, billowing like chiffon in the wind.

Movement.

EIGHT

1997
One Snowy Night

If someone were to ask what I've been doing the past seven years I might answer, 'easing myself through the gates of acceptance.'

When I first became unwell I was certain of some degree of recovery. At the age of thirty seven – after many years of studying and working toward a career – it was not in my nature to simply let go. Progress was slow but eighteen months into the illness my brain seemed to go into free-fall, burning up with thoughts and ideas as I lay in a semi-darkened room hour upon hour.

Energy wise – to be able to go anywhere – do anything – outside of my limited domestic routine, entailed resting up days before the event and then recuperating for days afterwards. The face of 'normality' I presented to the world, during any short excursion beyond the house, belied the degree of effort it took. But the weird, over-active energy coursing through my brain compelled me to think beyond this curtailed existence.

It often seems in trying to answer one question – in this case, 'How can I put some meaning back into my life?' we simply beget yet another question.

★ ★ ★

'Do you honestly think it's worth it?' Leopard quizzed me one snowy night a couple of years ago.

I replay the memory of that night bringing it into the present tense.

I am lying across some padded chairs in the Philosophy common room at the University of Warwick, where I'm enrolled as a PhD student. Attempting a research degree is the consequence of all that feverish brain activity – possibly not what the doctor ordered in terms of working towards a recovery. But this is the place I venture to every few weeks in order to touch base, attend the odd seminar and somehow convince myself I'm still part of the real world. It had seemed a good idea at the time and I'm clinging to the notion that it's preferable to be exhausted and mentally satisfied, than exhausted and mentally frustrated.

Leopard knows better – but he also accepts I'm stubborn in the face of defeat. The car journey alone is taxing – then I have to be careful to park near to the entrance of the Philosophy block because I'm unable to walk more than a few metres. Climbing the stairs is like tackling the steep ascent to a mountain top. But somehow – when I'm settled in (this is after all the familiar department where I completed my undergraduate studies ten years ago) I feel at ease. For the space of an hour or two I can be me, beyond the illness, beyond all the restrictions and it simply feels good. But then there's the backlash.

I'm shivering and huddle down, muttering under my breath, 'don't mither me Leopard – it can't be helped that the car won't start!'

The car breaking down means I've been away from home – from my bed – far longer than I can physically sustain. My body and brain are protesting and any ability to stay upright is rapidly deteriorating. The wait for the RAC rescue service has become problematic and I just want to be safely on my way. The snow falls in drifts, a pretty sight from the window which looks out onto a lit courtyard with pergolas and trees, but I'm fearful the roads must be icy.

'I used to be braver than this,' I whimper, thinking back to difficult commutes out of London – the time when I had to drive down the motorway in freezing fog with broken windscreen wipers – and the terrifying incident when I dodged a crazed driver as she careered down the wrong lane, driving straight towards me at high speed.

I curl up tighter when a friend brings a cup of tea. I hope she leaves soon because I don't want her to see me crumble. I don't want anyone to see me crumble.

How am I going to get home and what will I do when I get there? My son and daughter live independent lives now and Matthew is working in London. There's just me and the cat at home. Well – me and the cat and Leopard.

Matthew finds it strange being away – has never fully adjusted to the emptiness of our little flat – with my room just as it was when I worked there – the space frozen in time because I've never been back. A lone bottle of Musk bath oil remains in the bathroom cabinet and the floral pattern I painted round the mirror one night, when I couldn't sleep, is gradually fading – all the bright colours bleached out to faint pastels.

'It's only a minor mishap,' the RAC mechanic kindly informs me. 'You hadn't turned the ignition key correctly'.

I am mortified – how could I have been so daft?

'Am I allowed to ask you again?' Leopard ventures.

'Go on then – you're not going to let me off the hook 'till you do.'

'Is it worth it? The effort it's taking to engage with this philosophy *stuff*?'

'You think it's just *stuff* then?'

'I'm not going to answer that one for you – you need to work it out for yourself.'

NINE

1999
The Long Sleep

There are moments when I feel I've been bewitched into a deep trance; that one morning I'll simply open my eyes and become fully conscious, realising the past nine years have been nothing but a long, lingering sleep.

Nine years – I still track this state of being through accepted notions of time.

'How long?' people ask, and I count the years on my fingers, mentally clocking 1991,92,93,94,95,96,97,98,99 …

'How long have you been laid up?'

'Eight fingers and one thumb!' a small voice replies.

I can see the child now, my four-year-old self, sat on a tiny wooden chair at a desk. The child's mother is standing in the doorway to the classroom – smiling and waving goodbye. The little girl begins to cry but then notices the desk is covered with plastic shapes, consisting of squares, triangles and circles – each with a hole in the middle. Concentration and a quiet determination take over from anguish as she threads the shapes onto a piece of string.

Then – she grasps an abacus. '1 2 3 4 5 6 7 8 9!' her small voice boldly enunciates in perfect time with the brightly coloured beads flying across the piece of wire. The child is triumphant in her mastery of ordering the world.

How many apples, dogs, cats, chocolate biscuits, pieces of toast?

The experience of numbering, collating, builds a necessary survival skill. Life begins to revolve around structure and the structure that once made us feel secure becomes the straightjacket we call responsible adulthood. Removing the straightjacket is scary, even though it means a kind of freedom. I have felt so afraid of the mental freedom my illness confers, stripped – as it is – of any physical counterpart.

To enter the front rooms of the house before 9am is unsettling and I must wait until the hum of traffic, and the laughter of children making their way to school, eventually distils into a neutral silence.

I remember the thrill of a freshly washed school uniform, the red gingham crisp against my skin and my long hair neatly plaited and accessorised with matching ribbons and hair slides. As a child every new day felt *exciting.*

By 9.30am, I usually return to bed with a cup of tea and drift into sleep. It is so very difficult to stay awake. The sound of children's laughter fills my head and my vision is drawn towards the flickering sunlight on the bedroom wall as it projects a filigree lace pattern.

Leopard settles down on the end of the bed but he is a

little agitated. He senses a preternatural energy in the room and the flickering induces a hypnotic spell.

Memories stir as we fall into a semi-conscious state and the child, who a moment before played with the abacus, waves at us to follow her through another portal of time.

★ ★ ★

The year is 1956, and it is several months before the memorable day when the child experiences her first morning at school.

Just now, she is excited because a new family has moved into the avenue and she has made friends with another four-year-old called Lisa. The little girl enters the child's world with a flash of light bouncing off bright red curls and an aura of energy that seems to draw strength from a magical source, which the child's mother defines as *waywardness*.

The four-year-olds become inseparable and the child discovers a delicious, vicarious pleasure in watching the naughtiness of her playmate. This way – she avoids incurring the displeasure of her own mother who always maintains she can take *her* girls anywhere. With her older sister at school all day the little girl's loneliness is salved by Lisa's presence.

In the summer months the children play out of doors and their favourite game is witches, but in the autumn they mainly set up camp in the child's bedroom. Once they begin school their home playtime is restricted to weekends.

The novelty of the bedroom isn't to be found in the collection of teddies and dolls, or the bed with the saggy mattress that makes a great trampoline, or even the large empty cupboard which is big enough to hide in, but an old black gramophone player and a collection of 78rmp records. The records are mainly classical – but this suits the children as they spend their entire playtime swooning around in old lace curtains whilst dancing to the music. Their favourite game is pretending to be swans in the ballet Swan Lake. Lisa has seen pictures of the ballet in her Princess comic and now it is all talk between the two girls of wanting to be ballerinas. Here in her bedroom, amidst her mother's old net curtains and records, the child's ambition is born.

For a couple of years the ambition is easily satisfied by the dressing up game. Besides, the child's mother has other ideas. The ordeal begins at the age of six. The six-year-old knows that her mother loves to play the piano and admittedly the calm that descends on the house when she does so is wonderful – but the little girl's own efforts at this particular skill are to no avail. The weekly piano lesson is a dreaded ritual. It's hard to decide which is worse – either the teacher, an elderly church organist who smells of moth balls and mercilessly works her fingers crazy with endless series of chords – or the trauma of getting to the lesson? The child only has to walk to the bottom end of the avenue to reach her teacher's house, but every footstep feels perilous as clocks are adjusted and the dark winter nights set in. Every shadow cast by the street lights, every little mew of a stray cat – or a dog's sudden bark – makes her jump.

When Lisa enrols at the local dance school a plan is hatched. At the age of seven the child swaps piano lessons for ballet. She is jubilant!

The ballet teacher, with hair that is an odd shade of orange – not a vibrant red like Lisa's – has a temper that instills fright if not respect. However – she declares her new pupil is a natural. Lisa is not so fortunate and has decided straight off that this haughty ballet teacher is not someone she's bothered about pleasing. The teacher has found her match in a reluctant young girl who refuses to observe the niceties of the correct way to tie the ribbons on her ballet shoes or tidy her hair neatly underneath the obligatory pink headband. Lisa's white tunic hangs in creases despite her mother having washed and starched it the previous day.

'Lisa – don't you care about doing things properly!' the ballet teacher thunders.

Lisa has a particular 'look' when confronted by people in charge who she doesn't like. The child secretly admires her friend's courage and insolence – it's an attitude she never dares. Lisa doesn't stay the course but the child knows she must stick it out if she is to be a dancer.

'There's no short cut to being a ballerina …' she reads to her disinterested playmate from a new Princess ballet book.

Lisa pulls a face. She is rapidly outgrowing everything she perceives as childlike. In many ways, this adventurous seven-year-old is responsible for hauling her more cautious friend into the temporal world.

'But Lisa – I really do have a fairy in my bedroom,' the child protests. 'I can see her when it's dark and what's more she makes a tinkling sound so I always know when she's near.'

Lisa scoffs at her friend – not having read Peter Pan she's unaware of the plagiarism and simply thinks her playmate is dotty. She wonders if it's something to do with the little girl's blond hair – which is always beautifully brushed out and held with a hair slide or pretty bow. There's something fairytale-like about her friend, so of course she'd be full of silly stories. Lisa takes pleasure in pricking the bubble of her playmate's imaginings – she laughs at the idea of resident fairies and teddies that talk, and worse still – magical dolls which disappear to another world through a time capsule made from an old cardboard box.

'You're telling lies. I'm going to tell everyone you're a big fibber!'

The child knows Lisa has power over the other kids in the street. Scared of being teased she runs upstairs to don tartan trews and pumps.

'Ok Lisa – you win, let's go play hide and seek.'

★ ★ ★

Leopard stirs and turns over as my mind flits back and forth in time.

My body shudders as I fall deeper into sleep and each breath strips away another layer of time. It's like holding down the rewind button on a video film.

Between the age of seven and fourteen, ballet was all I really wanted to do but the enthusiasm eventually fizzled out. In my early teens I had a sudden inability to stretch my feet and point my toes without excruciating cramp. I experienced this as a failure and was too ashamed to tell anyone.

In the intervening years Primary and Secondary school became an anxiety provoking game of academic snakes and ladder.

★ ★ ★

The eight-year-old hands a report card to her mother and a school photo. The school photo is of more concern to the little girl. She doesn't understand why her mother suddenly had a thing for short hair. Gone is the long blond hair, bunches and plaits. It's true she still has the odd ribbon bow or her fringe clipped back in a hair slide (she could not have relinquished her Scottie dog hair slides) but she doesn't quite recognise herself anymore.

'Well done dear,' her mother encourages as she reads that her daughter is *'a little unsure of herself, but very well behaved'*. Her Class position is 27 out of forty children.

Four months later the little girl has climbed the ladder to position 16, and continues to be described as *'a very well behaved child.'*

By the age of ten she's slid down to position 25 – but her conduct is still *'very good'*.

On reaching the age of eleven – her final year at primary school – the child thinks she must have thrown a double six and hurled herself up one almighty ladder to near top position in class. Her teacher writes in a final school report, *'she has made an 'all out' effort to improve her standard of work and this she has achieved. Her examination results are excellent. Conduct – very good.'* The child feels a little glow inside and thinks perhaps she will be joining her older sister at the local grammar school.

★ ★ ★

The two sisters sit in the back of the car during the long journey home from their holiday 'up North'. There is only one topic of conversation – the contents of the brown envelope that will be waiting in the hallway with the rest of the mail.

'Don't worry if you haven't passed,' the child's sister comforts, 'it's too posh and the teachers can be really strict. You probably wouldn't like it and all your friends will be going to another school.'

But on opening the envelope the conversation has to be reversed.

'Oh – well done! You'll have a great time and I'll be there to keep an eye out for you.'

The child knows she will have only one year of older sister protection to rely upon but she figures it will be fine. The only drawback with having a big sister at the same school is that it will mean more hand-me-downs. Her mother must have reckoned on this because she has kept *all* of her sister's old school uniform!

The eleven-year-old is beginning to grasp that life is continuous change. The year of her ninth birthday there had been a new baby sister. The baby's head sprouted tufts of strawberry blond hair (though Lisa had insisted it was red).

'I'm going to form a club,' she'd grinned, 'for all us redheads – 'cos I think we're pretty rare.'

The arrival of the new baby heralded an era of wealth. The blue piggy bank – one of the child's treasured possessions – usually rattled with the odd penny, but for the first year of the baby's life it was regularly filled with threepenny bits.

Every time the baby cried – which was quite frequent – the child's mother would get a headache.

'If you give me a head rub you can have threepence to

spend,' her mother pleaded, in a tone of voice pitched higher than the baby's cries.

Or, 'Take your sister for a walk in her pram and you can have threepence to spend on sweets.'

The little girl was good at saving her pocket money, but sometimes she and Lisa could not resist the temptations of the sweet counter and sat on the kerb side counting out their stash of penny chews, gobstoppers, sherbet dabs and aniseed balls.

Since reaching the age of eleven the two friends have been allowed to walk up town. The route takes them up a steep pathway the child's mother refers to as 'the bank', which leads past a Catholic church. Sometimes they take a short-cut that runs directly alongside a convent which is partially hidden behind a high wall. The children run past the wall laughing and joking – glad they're not locked up the other side with the nuns who wear strange looking clothes.

In town they make a bee-line for Woolworths. The child always ends up buying her baby sister a toy. The baby has become a cute toddler who follows her around and wants to play. The child is quite resolute within herself; she would rather have a real baby sister than a lifeless doll which she has to breathe magic into. Once, she had even stuck a nappy pin into one of her doll's legs – not hard – but enough to see if there was a response. She feels bad about it now – she would never stick a pin in her baby sister!

It's true that some days her mother is more tired and grumpy and her father has to help out. Helping out doesn't seem to bother her father one little bit. The child thinks her dad isn't like the other fathers in the road. For a start he doesn't have any 'vices'. By that she understands he doesn't go to the pub. Her father would never do that because he's taken something called 'the pledge' with her mum. But when nana and granddad come to stay they go for trips out and stop off at a pub and she has a bottle of pop in the back of the car, while her little sister slugs cold tea from a baby's bottle – which doesn't look nearly so nice! She thinks her father probably drinks fizzy pop too but nana says he should have a bottle of stout because it's full of iron and will do him good.

Nana knows all about drinks that contain iron (the eleven-year-old isn't quite sure how iron gets into a drink and thinks she'd better ask – in case the question comes up in one of those increasingly difficult general knowledge tests her teacher keeps handing out at school).

She's gathered there's Sanatogen wine and Sanatogen powder that you have to mix with water – but that looks horrible – like chalk that's been all crushed up. The wine smells nice though and sometimes nana pours some into a little glass and lets her have a sip.

The child has noticed that granddad drinks something very different. It's dark brown and when he pours it from a bottle it's all creamy and frothy at the top of the glass. She can tell when granddad has drunk more than one glass at the pub because his face is red when he comes home and he's very jolly and always wants to sit and smoke loads of tabs and tell lots of stories.

The best story is the one about when he fell in the docks. Granddad has a favourite pub 'up North' – near to the docks, and he calls in there most evenings. Nana never knows what time he'll be back for his tea or who he might bring with him.

Sometimes he even brings stray animals home. Well one night – a long time ago – he was a bit wobbly. The child has noticed the brown drink does make granddad unsteady on his feet – though he still manages to dance on the table and empty his pockets of all his coins. This is a good thing because the next day she gets to travel on the train with nana to Newcastle and can spend her pocket money on whatever she likes. Anyway, one night granddad fell in the docks and was in the water all night 'till a policeman helped him out and took him home to nana.

That story was about a time before the child was born. She thinks her granddad talks about the past a lot – particularly the time he met nana. Her nana was the prettiest young woman he had ever set eyes on – with lovely brown hair right down to her waist. The child knows this is true because she's seen a photograph of her grandmother, with a plait so long it disappears off the edge of the picture.

When the family are on holiday 'up North' they all walk down to the docks and have a glass of lemonade at granddad's favourite pub. He's been going there for years and seems to know everybody. The little girl loves the walk because it cuts through a wood yard and she and her little sister play hide and seek and rabbit spotting amongst the wood piles. The pub is down a little alleyway just off the water front. The water in the docks is deep and murky and the child thinks maybe that's why her mum doesn't want her father to ever go to the pub when they're back in the Midlands – because it would be scary if he fell in some water and what if a policeman didn't come along – he might drown!

The child loves her granddad because he's funny and

knows magic tricks like making pennies stick to the kitchen door without any glue but she's glad her dad is different again. So – maybe Lisa's dad is the one to turn to when maths homework proves a puzzle, but the child is certain none of her friends' fathers get up early on their free Saturday morning to see to breakfasts and housework. Dad woke her up with a breakfast tray of porridge followed by bacon and eggs and he could be heard whistling and singing and clunking about with the vacuum cleaner downstairs … and when she was off school with tummy ache he brought a boiled egg and a glass of milk upstairs during his dinner hour and made her laugh with a joke. Her father always cycled home at mid-day – even though it only left a short while for his dinner.

Sometimes her father disappeared for a couple of hours and came back a bit muddy with his football kit. This is another thing that makes him special – he's good at playing football and doesn't mind at all that she's a girl and has even taught her to be goalie and how to head the ball. There's a glass display cabinet in the sitting room at home and every time her father wins a cup or a shield it takes pride of place on the top shelf. The other shelves contain a Coronation tea set and some little ornaments from their holidays 'up North'. There's a tiny teapot with the words Berwick-upon-Tweed painted on the side and a seagull stood on a rock. The seagull makes the child think of the beach and an exciting game of jumping over the waves she loves to play with her dad and little sister.

By the last term of primary school the two friends are beginning to feel more grown up and one day they make a dash for the make-up counter in Woolworth's rather than the sweets and toys. The child has already studied her older sister getting ready to meet her boyfriend, explaining to Lisa in great detail that 'getting ready to go out' involves much fretting with eye shadow, mascara and lipstick.

The younger sibling thinks the older group of teenagers look like film stars – especially the girls with their lovely, long hair (how did her sister manage that?) and their fashionable clothes (the fact of hand-me-downs was taking a more positive turn).

'One of my sister's friends looks like Elizabeth Taylor,' she informs Lisa, with a hint of pride.

It was true; the teenager was a beauty with her jet black hair and made-up eyes. She wore a cream jacket and skirt that neatly fitted a curvaceous body.

The child sighed – she simply couldn't imagine being that grown up.

'… and what's more Lisa – my sister has her own Cliff Richard's and Adam Faith records and she's allowed to use the new record player.'

The old gramophone had long died a death and her father ingeniously found a use for the ancient records by melting them down into plant pots with curvy edges. The child's record collection had diminished to a couple of Pinky and Perky EP's.

The younger children can't see into the future but a little further down the line someone significant is waiting in the wings. She is to become their idol. Friday nights will cease to be exciting because it's comic and sweets night – but because 'Ready Steady Go' is on the television and Sandi Shaw, with all her powers of attractiveness, will beckon to the heart of every teenage girl who is watching.

I track time by the changing patterns of sunlight on the bedroom wall. The patterns have disappeared when I open my eyes so I figure it must be late morning. The child has vanished into the ether but I'm left with my mind swirling with memories.

Within my memories the passage of time from childhood into young adulthood seems to pass imperceptively and Lisa and I have suddenly acquired long hair. I can't remember the steps in-between, when we graduated from one hairstyle to another in our quest for the Sandie Shaw look. Lisa reached this pinnacle far ahead of me and was generally more adventurous in her approach to growing up.

I attempt to wake from this tumble of recollections but a thought keeps repeating.

Impeccable conduct doesn't set the world on fire.

Perhaps it is the ghost of Lisa's spirit child whispering in my ear?

I never really learnt to let go of the need to please. An overt sensitivity was both my Achilles' heel and my strength – precipitating a tendency to throw myself wholeheartedly into tasks, goals and relationships. The problem with this is that energy may fail to flow in all directions equally and strength of passion in one area can leave a drought in another. I often burnt out trying to get the balance right and was no doubt occasionally annoying to others in the process.

In my adult life this tenuous balancing act was a recurring

theme until the alien situation of chronic illness took over and precipitated a monumental force of change.

Like time in reverse everything I'd worked hard to achieve began to unravel. A busy diary gathered dust and was eventually thrown away. On a more banal level the nice clothes – which I'd only just begun to afford – hung obsolete in the wardrobe. I had no need for a car because I was often too unwell to drive. In a bizarre way much of the materiality of life – beyond basic needs – no longer seemed a necessity. This was perhaps the starting point of seeking after a 'middle way'.

Even so, it was hard to abandon the plan to do further training to be a dance therapist. An enthusiasm for dance had been re-kindled – just months before I got sick – through participating in a series of dance workshops at the prison where I continued to work as a counsellor. We danced free style in bare feet – no tutus, stretchy tights and ballet shoes; no forced pointing – no cramping toes – nothing getting in the way of a wonderful sense of freedom. The impact of these workshops on the inmates was so positive that I knew I'd found a project I wanted to be involved with.

Following on from this discovery Matthew and I attended a couple of free-style dance workshops during which we threw our bodies around with abandon. We practiced at home – laughing and bruised – incredulous that we'd been taught to safely lift individuals heavier than our own body weight. Excitement!

In many ways, I guess I'd only just hit what might be considered the success lane when I became ill, but not long enough to be free of working class principles based on thrift. Just as well considering DWP benefit is not appropriate to middle class commerce. But I am lucky, incredibly fortunate, because of Matthew's care and protection. We keep our heads above water and have everything we require – apart from time.

Time – Matthew and I are apart during the working week and we hate it. Time has become the most elusive commodity of all.

TEN

What If?

What if the ongoing situation is truly a dream and I suddenly wake to a former life that turns out to be my real life – the one I had before all of *this* began?

How strange to leap out of bed and feel strength in my limbs; to run up the stairs and race from bathroom, to bedroom, to kitchen. How strange to have lunches to pack and housework to complete before dashing off to station or motorway – then to burn up the miles, sometimes with vigour and sometimes with weariness – because the journey was always there to be made, stretched out like an elongated umbilical cord joining work to home.

Before 'the dream' Matthew and I made the best of our split existence. Home in London was the basement flat mentioned earlier, not devoid of old-world charm having been untouched since the turn of the century. The kitchen, doubling as a therapy room and sleeping space, was graced by a Victorian stove – gathering dust. A service bell board hung on the wall – a reminder of servants long demised.

Our landlady, an elderly spinster of hearty, upper-class stock was installed on the top floor. Her female companion, a blind octogenarian of Polish origins and former aristocratic connections, lived on the floor below.

The house seemed divided into segments encapsulating past eras. Post-war, upper-class gentility was positioned on the top floor, whilst the floor below represented a microcosm of the cultured élite of pre-war Poland. Occasionally, our landlady descended from her attic room and her companion emerged from behind embroidered screens. We all met in the neutral space of the sitting room situated on the central floor, to sip sherry from cut glass.

Matthew and I were affectionately enveloped by this eccentric household. Ensconced in our basement flat, devoid of any amenities that could be classed as mod cons, we were not part of the Hampstead whirl.

In the semi-lit rooms, two in total, we made a cosy nest – with Matthew settled in one room and I in the other, and the flat gently humming with the emotions discarded by our clients.

Despite the cosiness there was a shadow and the shadow increased its power. The space began to close in as I worked and slept in that one room. If only I had realised what was to happen I would have ran. A primitive, animal instinct signalled flight but my human-self felt bound by a sense of responsibility.

Leopard fidgets – nervously; he has heard this story so many times and often reminds me I would have probably fled to another entrapped space – that life itself can become ensnared by the desire to escape a perceived entrapment.

Even so, there was something destabilising about our

lifestyle, not least of all the constant sense of packing and unpacking our belongings. I tried to get round this by having two of everything essential but the strategy didn't work in the area of essential emotions. Emotions resist the easy subdivision of pots and pans, toothbrushes and bars of soap. I missed my children on the days away from home and craved the normality of a settled routine.

Domesticity has the potential to make shape-shifters of us all. Princes become frogs and frogs become princes. Princesses may be awakened into life or numbed into a deathly unconsciousness by a kiss. A home may constitute either a fairy palace or a humble abode, or even (in the worse possible circumstances) a gloomy dungeon. By 1989, through the course of my thirty seven years on planet Earth I'd managed to shape-shift through several potential permutations – but finally I'd found stability with Matthew.

Leopard sighs at the gaps in my account.

'Well – there is so much of it,' I try to explain. 'What to include and what to leave out?'

Leopard remains silent. I am silent too – I want to see where the silence takes me.

'It's like this,' I finally say. 'Within the confines of this geographical space named home and garden – and through the events of the past nine years – I've embarked on an unplanned journey with no fixed destination.'

'A journey you didn't choose?'

'Yes – that's true. But this imposed situation has encouraged me to travel deeper into my inner world than I might have done because it was easy to pretend there was depth to my life before.'

'… and what about now?'

'Now there are no convenient terms to describe the places I've visited within the labyrinthine landscape of the mind.'

Leopard sighs. 'Tell me – why do humans have to so obscure?'

'I'm not trying to be obscure – but the only way I can describe this experience is to say I've discovered beautiful tourist hotspots where I've wanted to linger – but also locations of danger and unrest that few would voluntarily choose to include on their bucket list of places to visit before they die.'

'Of course none of this may be real,' Leopard challenges, 'it might all be a dream – or a nightmare – depending on whether you're having a good or a bad day?'

Will I be afraid to wake if this is just a dream?

How strange to wake to the sound of a fourteen-year-old Amy – to hear the tap-dance of Doc Martins as she feeds cats and rabbits before setting off for school. How strange to wake to the rhythmic beat of seventeen-year-old Stephen's music wafting downstairs – the prescient lyrics of The Wonder Stuff's 'Caught in My Shadow' – circling round in my waking thoughts.

Nine years on the house is silent – my children's teenage years long swallowed up by the passage of time. We both lost out and gained. I became the mum perpetually in her dressing gown, not capable of bearing much in the nature of discord or disharmony but still capable of love.

My perception was that I could never do enough and it is

true that intentionality always fell short of action. Worse still, the illness induced a short fuse when it came to noise. Even everyday levels of sounds such as kettles boiling: refrigerators humming: dishwashers slushing: raindrops pattering on the roof: planes passing overhead: dog's barking: the cacophony of televisions, radios and stereos, and the background hum of people talking, all magnified and disorientated my sense perceptions. Sound simply hurt and increased the head-pain and mental fatigue. It must have been a claustrophobic environment for two normal, energetic teenagers. For myself, this heightened intolerance to noise was an unnerving reminder of childhood memories of my own mother's inability to cope with any extraneous sound that lay outside her direct control.

Some might say that physical passivity is not necessarily harmful as long as it is wedded to emotional attention. I clung on to this comforting notion as I struggled to give out attentiveness from the murky depths of a totally fogged brain.

I look up at a photomontage of significant moments in Stephen's childhood. There are photomontages of both children in the study, so I am surrounded by their presence from babyhood onwards. There is a particular photo of Stephen's eighteenth birthday and I will never forget that day – for two reasons. Celebrating a young person's rite of passage into adulthood is a happy, memorable event – but sadly that day also marked the start of my illness. I recall setting candles and wrapping presents with a touch of flu. It was nothing terrible, just feeling a bit unwell – would be able to sleep it off the next day. *Sleeping it off* never materialised and our lives changed forever.

If I wake and find my present perception is only a dream could I allow myself the exhilaration?

Would I still be me, would Matthew still be Matthew, would Amy still be Amy and would Stephen still be Stephen? Or would we all be different characters in a totally new story?

The meandering gains momentum as my thoughts swirl off into a parallel universe where life is working out just as planned. Leopard opens his jaws wide and narrows his yellow-green eyes. Fixing me with a certain look he murmurs that the world of perfect plans is the illusion of the fool's paradise.

ELEVEN

Leopard's Poem

The process of meandering has become strangely illuminating and some might perceive my current status as the opportunity to live inside a gilded cage, from within which I'm fortunate to be able to spend time in reflective thought. So will I be content to relinquish the *privilege* if I wake to find the past nine years are merely the manifest content of a lucid dream?

In a parallel universe this passage of time is a mere blink of the eye. I receive a letter from a client who has not contacted me for some years. Her memory of our relationship is vivid and therefore startling. It's as though I have just left the room for a couple of minutes and all original attributes of vitality and human presence remain intact. I begin to cry.

'I don't want this!' I remonstrate. 'I want my life back.'

Leopard is agitated; his yellow-green eyes flash a look as though to say, 'Let it go, let the waters flow and don't resist the tide.'

'It's so hard,' I tell him. 'I want to dive into the ocean, to swim with grace and ease; I long to be strong – to be whole again.'

Leopard stretches. He turns onto his back and four heavy paws flop down.

'Remember,' he says, 'that holiday at Exmoor a couple of years ago? You told me you had stopped trying to get down to the sea.'

I think hard. All of my holidays with Matthew have blended into one memory that is inextricably cut down the middle, signifying a *before* and *after.* In the *before* half I'm swimming in a lake in France. The surface of the lake is covered with water lilies and the tendrils reach down below the surface and brush against my legs. I swim directly into Sun's rays; there is so much power and raw energy in my body that it's effortless to reach the far shore of the lake.

The *after* half depicts my lying on a day bed (two years later) loosely wrapped in a blanket. The blanket is pulled over my eyes to shut out the light – the only defence against searing head pain. This must make a strange sight because Matthew has made the bed high up on the moor, overlooking the bay. I tell him to take a walk through the heather and gorse because I cannot bear for him to be constrained

I have a recurring dream about needing to get down to the sea. In the dream I am restrained in a wheelchair and the sea seems to represent the essence of freedom. It's as though all would be well again if I could only take a walk down to the water's edge.

But Leopard and I have to figure things differently because the above train of thought only leads to despair. You might label our attempt to mentally survive as rationalisation, or you could be mean and talk about the construed payoffs of chronic illness, or you may decide to ponder (more kindly) on the degree of determination it takes to make something good come out of a difficult situation.

Whatever, the only way I can deal with what has happened is to go with the experience and try to extract some meaning I may not have been open to if my life had taken another course.

This has not made me a better person and that's the hard part. I have not become an infinitely compassionate human being – miraculously transformed (in some beatific way) by illness. Leopard scoffs at the idea of such a thought! No – it's the complete draining away of ego that interests and has become a subject of contemplation.

I lay on the day bed with Leopard at my side and he knew I was sad. It is miserable not to be able to walk on the moor, free to feel the wind on one's face and the bracken crackling under foot. Yet there is another part of me that is having a different experience. I have to mentally release this aspect from the painful physical sensations.

With eyes closed I sense a white light hovering above my body and feel a strong desire to join with the light. I stay with this pleasant sensation for a few minutes and on re-opening my eyes fix my vision upon a tree that has become permanently bent in one position. It's as though the wind only blows in one direction and the tree gracefully allows itself to be taken up by this current of air. I repeat opening and closing my eyes for several minutes.

In the background Leopard makes a rhythmic purring sound akin to a chant – a sound that also emanates from the white light. I am enveloped by the white light and the soporific cadence of chanting. I envision blurry human forms, shining with iridescence, and though I chide myself for such mystical notions I feel these semi-human forms inhabit a place called home – *my real home*. I am not meant to be lying on a day bed, draped in a brown blanket. My destiny is to become one of the iridescent creatures who have the magical powers to transcend human frailty and pain. For a few moments – even with my eyes wide open – the iridescent forms remain.

But my head fills with words and I feel I will never be free of words. Leopard instructs to listen hard because the words are the words of a poem and evidently poems can be particles of energy.

'Like particles of white light? I ask.

'Mmmm … white light is pure energy.'

Leopard's Poem

I lie still

Body-mind, sinks
into the purple heather,
emotions become a
mere ripple of grasses.

I lie still

The ocean flows within,
waves lap upon contours
of bone – the sting of sea-salt
penetrates soft tissue.

I lie still

Sound evaporates
into a whisper of air,
the trace of movement
is a droplet of water.

A single tear
reflected in
innumerable dewdrops,
calm now.

TWELVE

Riding the Starburst

I am not always calm. A particular kind of meandering precipitates a free fall into anxiety.

There is a process by which thought extends itself. Imagine a starburst gathering energy – with the energy of a starburst the mind creates and connects through memory and free association.

Once you get on the Starburst there is no knowing where the experience might take you. Accepted base camps like cliché and socially created systems of signs are passed by. You're on a one-way ride to the symbolic and living in the symbolic is an unsettling mixture of exhilaration and discomfort.

To live in the symbolic is to depart the safe, concrete world of material facts and to open oneself to what might be experienced as madness.

Leopard and I were dozing and on opening our eyes we saw Matthew standing by the fir trees in the garden, in the direct line of Sun's rays. I do not know which I registered first – sound or image? The loud, vibrational din of electric garden shears is an extended cutting sound lacking the speedy resonance of a quick snip.

My vision fixed upon a dark hole in the fir trees where Matthew had 'trimmed'. Within seconds the waving branches of variegated green had been reduced to a sad, empty space. I burst into tears, ranted, raved and snarled in protest.

The sight of the lacerated branches had triggered a chain-reaction, which gathered momentum at helter-skelter pace towards a mental image of severed hands. My mind was riding the Starburst faster than it could process the chaotic reaction to a seemingly innocent event.

Is madness a state of mind we get into when the imagination becomes distanced from reason? Applying pure reason to distress rarely seems to help to the same extent as unravelling the symbolic thought chain. Any form of art helps with the unravelling. Art and Literature are the means by which we ride the Starburst, the pathway to an understanding that consciousness is necessarily suffused with anxiety.

Leopard is edgy – his face clearly delineated by a look of feline concentration. He has a dislike for elevated categories such as Art and Literature. Leopard thinks more in terms of pictures and words.

'It sounds like a double bind,' he ventures. 'It's as though we can't understand anxiety without riding the Starburst yet taking the ride can produce the anxiety. Maybe life would be more comfortable if we remained at base camp?'

I try to imagine what it would be like to remain at base camp but the conjured image is of a blank piece of paper.

From as far back as I can remember base camp felt like an impoverished place to be. There was always another (supplementary) world of imagination; the concrete world was finite, static and boring.

The modern housing estate, where Lisa and I lived and played, was the important backdrop that circumscribed this other world. The estate had been built in the early fifties to cater for the exodus of workers from the North to the Midlands and represented a new way of life for families who had previously made do in subsistence accommodation. There was none of the bareness existing on many present-day estates. The wasteland my playmates and I frequented (which adjoined the estate) reverberated with rural opulence. We called this piece of land 'the bushes' because of the abundance of shrubs in which to play hide and seek. The bushes flowered and the trees shed conkers in autumn. The hedgerows produced handfuls of blackberries and I learnt my natural history from walks taken with my father over nearby fields.

Dad was a keen gardener and it seemed, in the playful world of childhood, that the roses were perpetually heavy with petals from which my friends and I made strange, perfumed concoctions.

These are the memories I try to retain, placed apart from the harsher realisations concerning adult relationships that children are inevitably exposed to.

A portion of what constitutes a happy childhood is essential ballast against the negative. The negative always exists waiting to pull us down, but learning to ride the Starburst is one way of dealing with emotional dark spots.

There are dark spots in my garden which cannot be

penetrated by Sun's rays. The dark spots are like the shadows in my mind – no place of comforting shade but an anxiety-provoking space.

'How serious you are!' a small voice scolds. 'Don't you know there are magic spells to get rid of dark spots?'

I think back to a time when my child's mind was full to the brim with magic but the spell eludes me.

'I can't recollect – please remind me.'

The child places a pocket mirror on the ground and drops a small stone from a height.

'There!' she smiles in glee, as the mirror shatters into several pieces.

The pieces are gathered and placed in a bucket which already contains pebbles and broken pieces of crockery. I spy Leopard asleep on the grass, sprawled out sunbathing. His back ripples and gently twitches indicating he is dreaming. In his dream, Leopard watches the child stride down the garden swinging the bucket.

The little girl wears a favourite sundress patterned with coloured circles and held by shoulder straps fastened onto bright, red buttons. Squatting down by a patch of dry earth she digs enthusiastically with a plastic spade. Small clods of earth fly into the air as the child digs and sings, lost in an inner world of schemes and plans.

Next, the contents of the bucket are emptied out and the pebbles neatly arranged in a circle forming a boundary line. The child inspects each piece of broken crockery in an attempt to figure some kind of unified image. She is uncertain whether the blue willow pattern markings suggest a segment of a bridge, or part of a bird's wing.

'La, la, la,' she sings. 'La, la, la!'

Leopard winces as the little girl pricks her skin with a jagged piece of mirror glass. She is only playing with danger but Leopard knows the single image is one of thousands that will attach to the symbolic thought chain. The image may lie dormant for a lifetime, never to be re-activated, or it may suddenly leap into life in a different and possibly more sinister context.

The child stands and surveys her work, then runs at a pace down the side alley leading to her father's front garden. The garden is a profusion of flowers and she reasons it won't matter if she picks a bloom or two. Her small fingers pull at the pink and blue candytuft; then she scoops up a handful of fallen rose petals and neatly pinches the head off a peach poppy. Now it is time to skip, because it is boring to move in the same way all the time.

'La, la, la,' she trills, skipping back to her patch of earth.

The candytuft and poppy are arranged in a meat paste jar, reminding the child she is hungry, and in a final exuberant gesture the rose petals are thrown in the air.

'All finished,' she concludes.

'These days, nothing gets finished,' I inform Leopard.

'Hmmm …' he replies, without opening his eyes, 'that's because you still haven't learnt to stay in the dream.'

THIRTEEN

The Big Question

There is a time when we stop playing (which is to step out of a most important dream) and feel compelled to ask 'the big question.' This question is broached in terms of four simple words.

'And what would they be?' Leopard asks.

'What – is – the – point?'

'Mm… four words sure enough – but that's the sort of question only a human would ask.'

'Then let me get on with addressing my human audience Leopard.'

'Ok – there's no need to get tetchy!'

If you think back over your life you will probably be able to identify the instance when you stopped playing. This moment in time may seem like an insignificant event to others yet it becomes pivotal in the story of who you are.

Some of us are protected for quite a while from 'the big

question'. Religious belief is a high voltage protector and there was a lot of religion around in my family. I incorporated the idea of angels, higher beings and a place called heaven into my psyche fairly early on.

The notion that there were friendly, invisible beings looking after my welfare helped to ward off the anxiety evoked by 'the big question' well into my childhood.

'We've only reached the point in the story when you're eleven,' Leopard interrupts, 'so what happened next – did the friendly beings just disappear?'

'No – it wasn't quite that brutal. But if you want me to go on with the story Leopard you'd better get comfy because it takes quite a while for a child to grow up.'

Leopard sighs. 'You know – I wasn't a cub for very long. You humans really drag things out.'

'Well you'll just have to be patient – and though I don't want to be tedious I should probably begin by saying that being an adult in human terms doesn't *necessarily* equate with being grown up.'

Leopard gives me a withering look. 'Well – am I allowed to interrupt as you go along?'

'Sure – it's a bit like talking to the wall when you don't.'

A STATE OF CHANGE

The child has grown and the red gingham dress is replaced by dull beige, the house colours of Curie. The child would prefer to be in Nightingale (lime green) or Bronte (gold). In winter she is cajoled to wear a navy gabardine mackintosh and an oversized velour hat. The hat irritates as it blows off her head in the slightest breeze. Worse still, the rim has a badge embroidered with mysterious Latin words.

A strange domain of pageantry has usurped the safe world of primary school. A woman with silvery hair, tightly swept back into a bun, rules the new domain. Each morning, this dignitary glides down a long aisle (her subjects stood dutifully at either side). A voluminous black cloak billows in the menacing figure's trail.

The child murmurs to herself that she has always known witches are for real. Gathering her cloak about her the woman solemnly climbs the steps leading onto a stage and walks to the lectern. In a high trilling voice, modulated with perfect vowel sounds, she addresses the assembled as 'young ladies'.

Young lady? The child wonders what it is to be a young lady. She never quite gets it right. There will be a downward slide as the transgressions mount over the years but just for now good conduct does not immediately fall by the wayside. It is the academic game of snakes and ladders that's causing most concern. Things started out well enough, but by the second form six F's scrawled across her report card doesn't bode well. There is talk amongst the staff of her re-doing the year – the suggestion being that having an August birthday makes the child the youngest class member and she maybe needs time to catch up with her peers.

The embarrassed pupil is not happy with this plan and decides she must simply try harder. After all – she's thrown a double six before, caught up and won the game.

But this game is proving tricky. By third form the thirteen-year-old is at least climbing all the popularity ladders.

She is very happy with her friendship group and is described by the form teacher as *'a helpful member of class'* who has been voted in by the other pupils as Form Prefect. By fourth form this has been expanded to *'a pleasant and conscientious girl and a very helpful member of class.'*

The fifteen-year-old is worried. She wants to find a balance between being seen as 'nice' and an inward certainty that she's actually a bit of a rebel. She reckons some of the teachers have rumbled her but on the whole the tag of niceness is sticking. A few petty misdemeanours start to build to even out the balance, such as – not wearing a hat – detention: sporting white ankle socks in assembly – detention: painting nails in class – detention: flaunting jewellery – detention.

Regarding niceness, by the lower sixth she hits the jackpot with *'gay and likeable'*, but a term later this is balanced out by the same teacher noting, *'work is improving but her attitude should show a readier acceptance of work discipline'*.

The next stage of reckoning is the event of being voted in as a sixth form prefect – an acceptable point scored for niceness, which is then perfectly counter-balanced by her headmistress seemingly deliberately jabbing her with the pin of the prefect badge during the award ceremony.

'I hope you're going to show a greater sense of responsibility,' the headmistress hisses under her breath as she jabs the pin through the errant schoolgirl's thin jumper. 'I hear you were late this morning – and without your hat.'

For a moment the teenager locks eyes with the headmistress. The woman's eyes are piercing and must have once been of the brightest blue. There is a twinkling that has not clouded with age and the teenager detects a hint of mischievousness that has the potential to swiftly morph into a cutting look. There is a whole life-story within those eyes and for a fraction of a second the teenager sees a tiny speck of her own life reflected within this woman's gaze.

The headmistress smiles for the benefit of the assembled audience and the teenager sweetly smiles back. She is thinking about the planned sit-in she intends to take part in with some of the more politically minded students. The protest wasn't of any earth-shattering importance – being merely a trivial issue concerning pupils not being allowed to wear scarves of any other colour but navy and powder blue – but in this strict school fighting for small changes entailed quite a struggle.

'Oh well,' the teenager thinks to herself, 'learning to rebel has to begin somewhere.'

The teenager thinks back to a matter of greater importance that she'd had to attend to before rebellion could truly be taken up. It was the issue of religion.

The sixteen-year-old has a memory of when all *that* began. She had been just four years of age.

She recalls her father holding her up to the light of a beautiful stained glass window in a room within a building she'd christened 'the House on the Hill'. Her father had smiled at her words. In order to get to the room he had to push open a heavy wooden door. The building was in fact the Catholic church she and Lisa would regularly walk past on their trips up town in later years, but as a four-year-old the child was unaware of the significance of the building or the distinction between her parents' spiritual leanings (her mother having been raised a Methodist by devoted grandparents) and how this distinction sometimes brought stress into their lives.

The teenager recalls a mysterious man in a long black robe who regularly walked down from the House on the Hill to play piano with her mother and how, as a little girl, she couldn't understand why her mother spoke of the imposing figure as *Father.*

★ ★ ★

The little girl finds it all very confusing – surely her mother's father lives with nana? She is quite sure that her grandparents wouldn't like the man in the long black robe pretending to be an important family member and wonders if it would be best to tell granddad the next time they visited, or maybe she'd just mention the problem to nana.

What's more – she dislikes the garden attached to the House on the Hill. The man in the black robe isn't a tidy gardener. The patch of land is full of old stones that are written on and there are flowers strewn everywhere. Some of the flowers are half- dead and look brown and mouldy. Well – what was the good in that?

Granddad has a *useful* garden called an allotment. When she and her sister are on holiday they walk to the allotment on Sunday mornings to collect vegetables for nana, and if it's a sunny day granddad fetches the deckchairs from a little hut and they enjoy a picnic with fizzy lemonade and crisps.

'... and,' she wants to say to the imposter with the long dark robe, 'my granddad has a park! I'm not sure he's bought it but he has his own hut with a little black stove to keep him warm. There's a garden by the hut where he grows marigolds and cabbages but the rabbits come and eat the cabbages. They love them!

Granddad's very important because he looks after all the children who play in the park and if they fall over he puts a plaster on their knee.'

The child misses her grandparents. They live such a long way off – someplace called 'the North' and it means a tiresome journey. Once they'd travelled by steam train – and the little girl shivers just thinking about the wild beast with its shrieking, clanking and hissing – and clouds of dirty, smelly smoke. Her father had lifted her up and she'd buried her face in his neck. They now make the journey in a new car – all squashed in with two dogs, a rabbit and a budgerigar – and she and her sister have to suck boiled sweets for the entire ten hours and try not to be car sick.

★ ★ ★

Concerning the House on the Hill the teenager remembers how her four-year-old self also noticed there was a lady with a baby living there. The lady stood next to a raised bowl of water.

All these years later, the memory of being scooped up in her father's arms as they stood next to the lady, remains a physical sensation. At this exact spot, her father had dipped a finger into the bowl of water and proceeded to splash the cold liquid on her forehead. Her four-year-old self had known very well that she'd washed her face that morning but her father always looked so serious when he did this strange thing that she let it go without protest. The lady with the baby never showed any surprise and simply continued to stand very, very, still – in fact, she never moved at all.

'It's a statue silly,' her big sister told her.

Most important though, she was allowed to hold her necklace when they visited the House on the Hill. The pink beads were pretty and strung on a gold chain with a cross. One day there was a big row between her parents and her father flung the necklace unceremoniously into the rubbish bin – along with a medallion she always wore pinned to her liberty bodice.

★ ★ ★

The memory of the House on the Hill may be strong but the teenager thinks it's because the details of the final day of any important ritual stick in the mind. She had enjoyed the Sunday outing – which is how her four-year-old self had perceived the visit – because it meant time with her father.

The teenager recalls that after the row she never visited the House on the Hill again and how a weekly event called Sunday School became the new routine. The 'new house' was plain in comparison, though it had a high balcony where she and her big sister sat away from their parents – along with all the other children – before they trooped off to various classes.

As the years passed by her parents were buoyed up by the new wave of evangelism within the Methodist Church and seemed united in embracing this alternative family of fellow church goers and their simpler traditions. Right up and into secondary school the child had not minded the weekly commitment – in fact she had been keen and volunteered as head of Scripture Union at school. Even so, she is now a little crest fallen that the only subject she does consistently well in is Religious Studies.

The sixteen year old feels uncomfortable thinking back to how she'd dealt with the situation of no longer wanting to go to church. By the age of fourteen she'd determined to find a way to extricate herself and had written down some thoughts in order to prepare for a meeting with one of the church members who took a particular interest in her.

Mr Newberry, I am really very sorry because I know you've been extremely kind and taken an interest in me all these years – but I should explain that I don't believe in a God anymore.

I'm quite sure that Jesus no longer wants me for a sunbeam (and I'm beginning to find that little song quite irritating when I teach it to the younger children at Sunday School) so I'm sure you'll agree this means I'd be rubbish as a missionary.

I am very sorry because you were so pleased when I told you I thought I had a calling and we even knelt down on the floor to say a prayer – and you blessed me, which was nice of you.

I now believe it was all the years of collecting money for Sunny Smiles that misled me – the pictures of those little children in the orphanages in Africa really had an effect – and I wanted to help.

I'm worried I'm stuffing up my plans at school because as you might know my headmistress is a member of our church. I've watched her float down the aisle – just as she does in assembly at school – right down to the front where all the important church members sit. When she sees me looking after the younger children she gives this little smile and tilts her head. She never smiles at me like that at school – which is annoying.

The trouble is Mr Newberry, that tilt of the head makes me feel like she's looking down on me and that she knows, in a not very nice way, that my dad is sat at the back of the church – not at the front. Dad refuses to go to open evenings at my school – it's like he feels that teachers are people he's supposed to doff his cap to (he doesn't wear a cap actually). Dad says he doesn't feel comfortable round educated folks – which is silly because he's the best person I know and he has a responsible job and lots of people think well of him.

I'm scared that one day my dad won't feel comfortable round me 'cos I intend to get very educated!

My mum's gone a bit strange on me too. I know mum wants me to have a good education because she's said as much – and she made a big decision to send my sister and I to the lovely new primary school on our estate – when we were small – instead of the Catholic school at the top of the hill. That school lies behind a VERY HIGH brick wall! Just think – I might have ended up there and had to cope with being taught by nuns – which Mum says is sometimes scary because they are not always kind. Mum knows all this for sure because she has a whole shelf of books about scary people who've been unkind to children in one way or another.

Mum also says it was because she didn't want me and my sister to end up having lots of babies. I haven't quite worked that one out but she needn't have worried because I'm only planning to have two or three.

My mum is bright but she had to leave school when she was fourteen – same for my dad. But that doesn't mean they're not clever or don't think about things.

As you probably know mum is doing a special course to brush up on her nursing and midwifery and dad is now a foreman at the factory, so I reckon my parents have done well.

Take religion – mum once got very troubled worrying about t-r-

a-n-s-u-b-s-t-a-n-t-i-a-t-i-o-n. I hope I never have to learn a word that hard to spell again! Well – that's how my sisters and I ended up your side of the fence not the Catholic side, because even though mum went to classes with the Catholic priest she says she can't ever accept that the bread and wine in communion are transformed into ... well you know how it goes. I'm not keen on the idea of that either.

But how many people really care about that sort of thing? I expect they just take communion and go home to their Sunday dinner. It shows my mum is a deep thinker – and she often says that – usually when she's trying to prove a point.

Well – to be honest, I can imagine myself worrying about little details too – because I'm more like mum than she realises. Sometimes my head spins round thinking and worrying about things to the point I feel dizzy!

I've always had a worry list – I can remember the list going right the way back to when I was four.

First off was the fear about the mad axe man. He came to me in a dream after I heard mum and dad talking about a girl who'd been murdered. I was sitting in the back of the car with my big sister and when I burst into tears mum realised I'd been listening and tried to change the story. She said she'd got the details confused and it was just a story about a hungry man breaking into a farmer's house to steal food from the pantry. I knew she was making up the story and couldn't get rid of the knowing that there were bad men out there who hurt children.

The trouble is – once you've got THE KNOWING there's no going back to feeling happy and secure is there? Not unless you use a bit of magic.

I'm afraid the revelation caused me to be quite anxious when I was little. Mum and Dad did their best to reassure me. Once Dad had to come and fetch me from the Work's Christmas party 'cos I started

*fretting about a lump in my throat. Even the jelly and ice cream –
which I'd been looking forward to – wouldn't go down and I thought
I was going to choke!*

*And then there was the time when mum got really poorly and was
whisked into hospital in an ambulance. I was only five and I thought
she had died because she was missing for weeks and children weren't
allowed to visit. Luckily, my friend Lisa's mum found me sitting on
the doorstep after school one day. She made me pink blancmange with
hundreds and thousands on top and kindly explained that mum was
getting better and would be home soon. And she did come home – but
no one explained that she had lost a baby – and had suffered something
called an ectopic that can be very serious and it nearly killed her. I wish
I'd known because mum was really quiet for a while and I thought it
was something I'd done to make her cross – and I can remember
wondering why she didn't smile when I gave her the colourful picture
I'd made with some new crayons Lisa's mum bought for me.*

*Anyway – things got back to normal and if I ever felt frightened I
would get into mum and dad's bed and mum had this story she used
to tell me. It was a very calming story about a beautiful garden that
had lovely flowers and butterflies and bees – and when she stroked my
forehead it felt like butterfly wings and I used to fall asleep real quick.*

*But I knew from being quite young that the world wasn't really a
beautiful garden – not when there were people in it – because people
were capable of doing horrible things. I was quick at learning to read
so by the age of nine I'd sneaked into mum's room several times and
read bits from a few of the books on that shelf designated for nasty things
that go on in the world. The books were a mix of religious topics and
war books. I must have been the only kid in the whole school to be
fully acquainted with the details of the holocaust at a young age.*

All of that really played on my mind and one detail played over and over. I'd read about a new born baby being thrown into the burning furnace of an oven. It was shocking because the story was about REAL life – not a Grimm's fairy tale of Hansel and Gretel. As if it wasn't already bad enough that my granddad had lost his arm in a different war! Granddad used to scare my big sister and me silly by fetching his prosthetic arm out of the back of the wardrobe. He'd fling the disembodied arm about and make fun of it – but really he was in a lot of pain where his arm used to be. He called it a phantom pain and tried to explain it was a pain you got when part of you had been taken away but your body tricked you into thinking it was still there. Granddad's body still wanted his arm because it shouldn't have been taken away and now he has an invisible pain – because nobody can see it – but that doesn't mean the pain doesn't exist or that he's making it up.

I sort of understood what he meant because sometimes I thought my mum had a phantom pain inside her head and that she hurt in a place where she shouldn't have hurt because something had been taken away – like the bit of your mind where you store all the nice things that have happened so you don't get really downhearted or annoyed. Granddad told me that his brother had been killed in the war and I thought in that case granddad must have that phantom pain in his head as well, and maybe my family was a little bit difficult at times because everyone was walking round with a phantom pain in their head for one reason or another?

When my little sister was born she was so tiny and vulnerable and because of all that worry rattling around in MY head I felt very protective of her.

Anyway Mr Newberry – what I was trying to explain is that once you've got THE KNOWING there's no going back to feeling safe and secure is there? For a long while saying my prayers helped but now I feel that's just another belief in magic.

I wish there was such a thing as magic. The first spell I'd want to try is one to make me more intelligent so I didn't have to struggle so much at school.

Dad always makes a little joke about me being the brainy one in the family. He looks at me and laughs and says, 'I don't know where you get your brains from – it can't be me,' which is plain silly, because if he went to an open evening he'd soon realise I'm not at all clever and I nearly had to repeat a whole year in second form.

Where do brains come from anyway?

So really, all I want to do just now is study hard and have fun with my friends.

(Oh … and find a good looking boyfriend. There are no good looking boys at church Mr Newberry and I need to widen my horizons!)

★ ★ ★

The sixteen year old recalls how she'd only felt able to say a fraction of what was in her mind. As she'd feared, the response of her church mentor was crushing but she knew she'd done the right thing. Walking away after their meeting the air on her face felt cool and clear. Then, a mental shackle dissolved as she felt a little tremor of excitement and anticipation. Now she could begin to explore who she really was!

The sense of elation was short lived. From some unknown place there came a physical jolt and the realisation that freedom is actually quite anxiety provoking. Freedom meant allowing a layer of protection to fall away.

… and there lay another item to go on her worry list.

★ ★ ★

The seventeen-year-old peers from behind a duffel bag strategically placed on her desk and stares discontentedly at the mole on her English teacher's face. The teacher is small in stature, with wavy grey hair clipped back with a kirby-grip. Everything about the teacher is dull – from the muddy brown crimpolene skirt (neatly cut – just below the knee) to the thick beige stockings which disappear (along with tiny feet) into clumpy brogues.

The subject of brogues was once a battleground between the teenager and her mother. To continue to wear brogues past the age of thirteen meant the inevitable, permanent slippage into *young lady-dom*. 'A fate worse than death!' she now muses, whilst wriggling cramped toes in pointed shoes.

The teacher is reading from Keats. She is in a paroxysm of adulation regarding the author's thoughts on beauty, love and eternity. The teenager feels a pang of sympathy. There is an accepted theory amongst her classmates that the cranky spinsters, who had landed en-masse at their school, had all lost lovers in 'the war'. There was no way at guessing the age of these women who had a style all of their own, so *which* war wasn't clear. The theory was a way of re-humanising the stricter teachers who lacked the saving graces of some of their more sweet natured colleagues.

Within herself, the teenager has decided there may be a connection between spinsterhood and the values of young lady-dom. She spreads her hand upon the desk and proceeds to paint a second coat of varnish on neatly manicured nails. There is a ring on her engagement finger; it has a small sapphire stone surrounded by tiny diamonds.

★ ★ ★

The seventeen-year-old and her friends are not accustomed to bothering with boys of their own age. Finding themselves in an all-girls school has resulted in the view that teenage boys are an alien species who fail to mature quick enough to be of any interest. The local engineering college provides a plentiful supply of older, better looking and more captivating potential boyfriends.

The teenager has already had her heart broken. She thinks back to the year of her sixteenth birthday when she spent the entire summer holiday with her grandparents, nursing the hurts of a love affair gone wrong and trying to work out why she had been rejected. With the naivety of youth she had determined this would not happen again.

It is always comforting to be at her grandparents. Her childhood memory of driving across the Tyne Bridge is one of passing through a final gateway to a beloved place and by the age of eight she'd learnt all the transitional landmarks encountered on the long car journey.

In the here-and-now of a warm summer's day, during a boring lesson, the teenager day-dreams about past journeys and holidays as her teacher's voice drones on in the background.

★ ★ ★

The old A1 road used to take her family to Doncaster which was the half-way point and here they all enjoyed a celebratory picnic to mark the event of leaving one world behind (the Midlands) and crossing the threshold to another (the North).

81

Deep in the North lay hills and valleys: rivers and streams: beaches and cliffs: rock pools and fishes and wild, purple-heather clad moors. The teenager remembers how the fun fair at Whitley Bay, exotically named 'The Spanish City', was a place of adventure. Here, as a little girl, she added to her list of Northern pleasures: rides on magical horses: eating sweet fluffy clouds called candyfloss: sucking on sticks of mint flavoured rock with writing inside 'till her tongue tingled and turned bright pink: the thrill of entering a room lit by flashing lights and filled with lots of tall metal boxes in which pictures of fruit spun round and round – before spewing out coins, *and* – most scary and exciting of all – chancing upon one special box, the home of a puppet policeman who came to life as he swayed to and fro, laughing loudly – 'ha-ha-ha-ha … hee-hee-hee!'

The first time she encountered the laughing policeman she clung to her father and asked if they could go outside and find the place where you could win a cuddly toy by pretending to be a cowboy and shooting a gun at some metal targets, or by hooking a plastic yellow duck from its little shallow pond.

When they arrived back at nana's – tired and hungry from their adventures, granddad would pull out the long wooden bench for them to sit at the table to have tea. As a child she had sat intrepid, rocking to and fro on the rickety bench, wondering what strange meal he would demand.

'Lisa – it's true – really, really true!' she insisted, on her return home. 'My granddad eats tripe – it's this horrible white stuff – with milk and onions.'

'Mmm … really?'

'Yes *really* – but much worse than that, he eats pigs' trotters!'

Lisa had shrieked with mock horror and the two young friends ended up rolling about on the grass verge.

'Pigs' trotters, pigs' trotters! Oink! Oink!' Lisa giggled in a squeaky voice.

As a child everything seemed different and fun at her grandparents – right from the moment she opened her eyes in the morning.

'Pop and cream cakes for breakfast,' she'd told Lisa, 'that's if there's any left over from the day before. And I don't have to have a proper wash because there's no bathroom.'

'No bathroom? Are you fibbing?'

'It's true – we have to take it in turns to wash at the kitchen sink – but granddad's got this new con …contraption – I think that's the word – that heats water, so nana doesn't have to keep filling kettles. You have to light it with a match and it makes a big bang!'

The teenager ponders how years later the Ascot heater continues to noisily whoosh and that it's still necessary to wash over the kitchen sink – but the magic of childhood is no longer there to protect her from her worries.

During the summer of her sixteenth birthday she had stood in front of the old dressing table in her grandmother's bedroom and wondered how to make the hurt go away. The dressing table is positioned by the window in the front room of the house and when she was small the room had seemed huge. It should have been the lounge but her grandparents preferred the back room leading onto the kitchen with its door onto a small yard.

As a little girl she had ran along the hall corridor towards that back room, with excitement and relief at being able to stretch her legs after the long journey. She was like a puppy dog gleaning the smells – the coal burning in the hearth, the odour of bacon and black pudding cooked in lard and the pungent trace of cigarette smoke and beer. Her grandparents were so happy to see them, welcoming the chaos of her family and accompanying menagerie of pets into their tiny home.

A small, moth-eaten monkey hangs on the dressing table mirror – it has always been there. The story goes that the child's older sister had brought the toy back from the fair when she was very small, and it was all that remained of her presence when the family moved to the Midlands. The child's older sister was the apple of her grandmother's eye because she had spent every day with her for the first two years of her life.

The front bedroom – though rarely used – contains most of her grandmother's treasures. The large double bed is always neatly made and her grandmother's best clothes hang in the wardrobe. The drawers contain neatly laundered linen; embroidered table clothes, sheets, pillowcases, cushion covers and curtains that are put away for another time. The mantelpiece is a display area for family photographs, the frames dated and labelled in her grandmother's spindly writing. There is an entire family history on that mantelpiece.

Another object the teenager thought her memory would always retain is the ornate chamber pot kept under the bed. She doesn't remember ever using the large yellow bowl with its gold painted rim but is sure she must have done as the toilet is quite a hike down the back yard. One of the things she likes about her family is that they are fairly uninhibited and despite the religious backdrop there is a down-to-earth sense of humour that flows with the rougher edges of life. This had enabled them to manage quite happily in the cramped space at her grandparents, apart from the odd family row when tensions arose that she didn't fully understand as a child.

But now, as she sits daydreaming in her classroom, she muses on how the tension eventually became like a dark, storm-filled sky and how she had gradually become part of the thunderclaps which intermittently broke into a more amicable atmosphere.

'Thunderclaps?!' Leopard suddenly snorts – sitting bolt upright. 'I'm not very keen on those. Are we going to have a storm?'

'Go back to sleep Leopard! I'm not talking about nature's thunderclaps.'

'Huh? You did say I could interrupt.'

'Ok – I'll explain what I mean. I think it might be best if I write it down.'

HOW THUNDERCLAPS ARE MADE

Person one makes a reasonable request or an innocent comment.
Person two gives a negative response.
Person one is upset by the negative response.
Person two expresses frustration that person one is upset.
Person one responds with escalating frustration.
Person two gets angry.
Person one retaliates or bursts into tears.
Person two is furious.
There is a big explosion of *noise*!

'Can I go on with the story now, Leopard?'

'Sure – but can I just say a biff on the nose usually sorts things out when leopards get annoyed with each other.'

★ ★ ★

In her sixteenth year, whilst looking at all the photographs on the mantelpiece, the teenager became aware that she held only tiny pieces of all the stories that might explain the stormy sky.

Just recently, she'd re-made contact with her dad's father – her distant grandfather, but sadly his wife – her barely remembered grandmother – had died.

The story went that the distant grandmother had once cradled the child in her arms at the event of her Catholic christening – which took place at the House on the Hill – an event the child's mother refused to attend. The teenager thinks this grandmother must have once cared for her if she'd come all the way from 'up North' just to hold her. She wondered – had her baby self cried at that first splash of holy water and had she been decked out in a white christening gown, all lace and frills? There was no photo so it was all conjecture.

Returning to the mantelpiece her eyes had lingered on her parents' wedding photo. Here were grandparents, aunts and uncles from both sides of the family, and she remembered meeting many of these relatives, but there had been a rift with her father's side of the family and the contact dwindled to the odd rare visit. The list of 'explanations' for the rift had always seemed arbitrary.

'There was no music at my wedding because I wasn't a

Catholic,' her mother proclaimed, in a tone of voice that clearly indicated perpetual annoyance.

'My father fell out with your mum over an unwashed porridge pan she'd left by the sink, when we briefly lived with my parents – just after the wedding,' her dad added to the story, 'so we came to live with nana and granddad.'

'Just think – we went all the way over on the bus to see them when you were little and got told to come back the next day because your grandmother was going out to play *whist*,' her mother continued, with a pained emphasis on the final word.

Whilst growing up, the child had heard mention of her distant grandmother's love of whist – how she played cards most evenings with her sisters, while her husband was away at sea working as a chief steward for the Ropener Company. A love of the ocean had overridden the injuries he had sustained during the First World War, and in his absence the social game of whist became his young wife's solace, along with a devotion to the Catholic Church. Meantime, her two sons amused themselves playing football by lamplight with their cousins and friends.

'I was brought up on jam and bread and dripping,' her father recounted – smiling, 'and my uncle looked after us a lot of the time.'

'Which uncle?'

'Uncle John – you remember – he had a hunchback because he fell down the stairs as a baby. He was such a lovely man.'

'Was Uncle John like mum's grandparents then?' she'd asked.

'In what way,' her father replied – puzzled.

'Mum always says her grandparents brought her up?'

The teenager remembers thinking that few adults in her family seemed to have been 'brought up' by their actual parents, and how the thought had worried her as a child because she didn't know who would look after her if a catastrophe were to happen. After all, she and her sisters were stuck in the Midlands with no grandparents, or aunties and uncles close by. It was thoughts like that which had caused the lump in her throat and sick feeling in her tummy from time to time.

'It's survival of the fittest in the jungle,' Leopard sleepily interjects, 'no friendly relatives there to give a hand.'

The sixteen-year-old had tried to put all the fragments together but it didn't really explain anything. Could an entire family really fall out over a porridge pot, a game of whist and a few clashes over religion?

Still ruminating, she'd walked to the corner of the bedroom to sit on the fold-out bed which she and her big sister had often squeezed into as young children – though sometimes they were expected to sleep next door at the doctor's house where a large, jolly lady they called Auntie Nora looked after things.

The teenager recalled how she'd hated the sleep-over because the house was big and creepy compared to her grandparents'. One night, she and her sister were allowed to stay up late and watched a series called 'Tales of Mystery' before going next door. The episode was all about spooky cats and had terrified her. She'd spent the entire night huddled under the eiderdown, afraid that dark shadows were coming out of an old wardrobe.

'You've got an over-active imagination,' her sister scolded, 'just go to sleep.'

Whilst stood in front of the dressing table at her grandparents', in the summer of her sixteenth birthday, the teenager had wondered if she was cursed with an overactive *everything*. She missed the ex-boyfriend with the beautiful long blond hair and an unfortunate predilection for drugs and suffered a physical pain when she thought about his cruel treatment of her.

Looking back now, in her seventeenth year, she acknowledges the relationship could never have worked because she doesn't comprehend the whole drugs scene. In her inner world, life is either intoxicatingly beautiful or unbearably sad. She can't imagine wanting to heighten her perceptions either way – her mind would simply implode!

During her stay the previous summer she had taken a fancy to a couple of items in her grandmother's wardrobe – a lilac dress with a little matching jacket and a long cream nightdress made from silk. The teenager thought the nightdress perfect for the local disco. Her grandmother – generous as always – said to keep the items along with a string of pearl beads. Once tried on, there was something magical about the nightdress. The teenager experienced a little shiver as she caught sight of her reflection in the dressing table mirror. She took home with her the realisation that she was no longer a child – gone is her innocence, gone is her belief in the perfect romance and gone is a piece of her heart.

★ ★ ★

Leopard stretches and gingerly gets off the bed. 'Mirrors are important to humans aren't they?'

'It seems that way – especially teenagers. Shall I continue?'

'Just remind me where we were?'

'In the classroom.'

'Oh yes – that sounds a very confined space; Leopard cubs wouldn't like that at all.'

★ ★ ★

The teenager continues to daydream about the past year as her teacher instructs the class to turn to a particular poem. She hopes she won't be asked to read from the poem because she's already been told – in so many words – that she's useless at reading poetry out loud.

The six weeks holiday, the previous summer, had brought about a positive change and put some distance between the sense of hurt at being rejected and the more recent excitement of becoming a sixth former. On returning home from her grandparents she had made the decision to have her hair cut short – Twiggy style. It seemed important to have a new image – a fresh start.

The daydream always reaches the same point of re-enactment as the teenager replays in her mind the night she first met her fiancé.

A few weeks after returning from her grandparents, not long after joining the lower sixth form, she'd gone with a group of friends to a local pub which was a popular meeting place. The girls were under-age but nobody seemed to care or even notice and it was easy to ask someone from the crowd to go to the bar and buy their drinks. Having tired of the new hairstyle she wore a long blond hair-piece – fashioned hippy style with a red headband and thought it looked very cool indeed with her grandmother's silk nightdress.

Her father had given his usual smile saying, 'don't know where you get your good looks from – it can't be me.'

She'd grinned, because it amused her that her father didn't seem to think he'd given her anything – brains or looks. It was all the usual silliness because he was quite handsome – better looking than any of her friends' dads.

The teenager visualises the room at the pub – a tiny space that's always crammed with people dancing, smoking, talking and generally having a good time. In their small town environment it's easy to sort out the locals from the influx of students at the engineering college. That night she'd stood apart from the crowd with one of her friends – deep in conversation – when two young men (clearly from the college) had walked over to them. One was blond with a cheeky smile and friendly manner. The other was dark and more reserved but the teenager recollects how she'd instinctively known he was the one for her. He was very good looking and now she has a photo of him slipped into her school folder – even her history teacher had asked to have a peek and whispered how nice he was. But that wasn't the draw – it was something about the eyes – the eyes had her.

★ ★ ★

The teacher enthuses further on Keats as the headstrong teenager continues to think back on the first meeting with her fiancé. The pupil feels certain she knows more of love, passion and beauty than the elderly spinster. This level of conviction is causing problems. She has pushed her luck in staying on at school because nobody expected a low achiever (by grammar school standards) to enter sixth form. And now she is whining on about studying philosophy. None of the staff at her conservative school seem remotely interested in the subject Philosophy – or if they are they're not letting on to this unlikely candidate. A pious R.E. teacher shudders at the very memory of philosophy students at her university.

'A weird bunch!' she proclaims, through a tight smile.

The pupil isn't considered bright enough by some of the staff to argue her case. She is categorised as an average student from an average background, hardly university material – but would perhaps make a nursery school teacher. Eventually a compromise is agreed. The average girl can apply to train as a social worker, and on completion can work for the good of folks deemed to be 'less than average' in every aspect of their lives. The R.E. teacher beams as she pronounces this 'excellent' solution.

The ambitious sixth former falls down a gap between convention and a slowly emerging new order. Younger members of staff are recruited and diplomatically work within the élite governance of the resident bluestockings, bringing a freshness and sense of modernity to the school. The sixth formers discuss fashion, boyfriends and even birth control with their younger tutors. One teacher is particularly keen for the teenager to apply for university and can't see any problem but the headmistress refuses her backing.

Even so, the sixth former cries on her final day at school.

For all its improbable lyrics and impossible high notes the school anthem brings a lump to her throat, and the raucous rendition of 'Jerusalem' renders the group of young friends speechless with laughter and tears. There is a degree of affection for this institution that has bestowed, in equal measure, the positive and negative aspects of a certain kind of education. Some of the female teachers will remain in the sixth former's heart as positive role models for young women and an eccentric old maths teacher (a subject she had remained rubbish at) was to prove a faithful friend in adult life.

Weirdness has the last word at the sixth form entertainment – an annual event put together by final year pupils. This event is popular simply because it's an acceptable format for making gentle fun of staff members – through sketches and mimicry. The teenager will have an abiding memory of her headmistress being persuaded to take part.

In the final scene of the performance the lights are dimmed for a few seconds. Suddenly – in the half-light – a figure comes running down the central aisle. The figure stops for a moment – caught in the glare of a spotlight. It is the headmistress – with … no … surely not … could this be for real? … with her long grey hair set free of its bun! The hair falls down the woman's back – the silver strands shimmering in the spotlight's glare as it tracks her frenetic moving image. The headmistress shrieks and pulls at her hair – she is a mad, crazy woman – she is a spectral incarnation of the fearful witch of the four, five, six, seven, eight, nine, ten, eleven-year-old child's imagination!

The image is superlative, stupendous – a memory to hold on to for life.

★ ★ ★

A few months later the newly emerged young woman is taking a Social Work degree and hating every moment. She falls asleep in lectures and yawns over Scientific American papers in the library. Her mind is sick of reading about monkeys, ducks and the whole idea of learning about human behaviour from animals. Something is very wrong as 'the big question' looms over her with ominous intent and nothing she reads is helping.

The young woman has just turned eighteen and soon the sixties will be a past decade. She reckons the hippy revolution has mysteriously passed her by with its incantations of free love and world peace and any opportunity to actually travel the world is well beyond her reach. She is working as an assistant cook at a local boarding school at the weekends, just to be able to eat and pay the rent on the house she shares with some fellow students. Her parents haven't quite got the idea of subsidising her grant and she would never feel comfortable asking them for assistance. Fortunately, her fiancé has a full grant and helps out.

Admittedly they had taken a holiday in Italy before she started college – which would have been frowned upon if they had not been engaged. But the abiding memory is of a hideous thirty-six-hour bus trip on a vehicle resembling a Midlands Red bus – except it was green. The Doge's Palace was surely memorable but they'd had a lovers' tiff and she had some moody photos to prove it, and – as she was terrified of pigeons – St Mark's Square was more like a scene from Hitchcock's film 'The Birds', than a place of architectural significance.

Then there had been a trip to Hyde Park to see The Stones in concert. She hoped this fact, along with the photos of her wearing a bright orange kaftan, would be enough to convince any future children that she wasn't a complete let down in the coolness stakes.

In her secret thoughts she conjures a dream of switching to a philosophy course someplace 'down South', where one polytechnic is offering the subject. It never occurs to think about applying to University.

The planned exodus 'down South' fails to materialize. A year later, by the autumn of 1971, a different path has opened up. Like multiple turns of a kaleidoscope the pieces of a life are continually thrown about to settle into new patterns. Often this feels random but whatever the shifting patterns the pieces remain the same.

For now, the pieces have fallen in a particular way and the young woman – soon to be a mother – sits in a damp room, where a strange variety of moulds adhere to every walled surface.

She thinks back to the summer months when the house had seemed adequate. After the wedding – and a holiday at her grandparents because there was no money for a honeymoon as such – it had been fun setting up home in what had once been her husband's student pad.

The wedding had been a lovely day. She'd worn a long Laura Ashley dress (bought during a trip to Carnaby Street the previous spring) patterned with tiny green flowers and had carried a yellow puff-ball of daisies. Her mother contained herself fairly well and there had been no histrionics in the morning. It had been a much bigger event than she'd imagined the previous winter, when she and her fiancé wondered about simply going to a registry office with a couple of friends. This thought had possibly been triggered by her discontent with her social work course and she had experienced, for the first time in her life, a sense of a lack of direction and a distinct low mood. She was now an auntie to twin boys and another friend had a sweet baby girl and the thought of babies was becoming a bigger pull than the mythical philosophy degree someplace 'down South'. She had not directly planned to be at the point she was now but there was a comforting inevitability about the situation. Marriage, babies and family she knew about – this other *thing* of stepping out of the mould was inexplicably wearing her down. How could it be that the one goal she'd been working towards since the age of twelve now seemed so disappointing? Was it that the course was wrong for her – just as she'd feared – or maybe that witch of a headmistress had been right all along and she simply wasn't bright enough?

But the day after the wedding something strange had happened at the train station as they waited for the train. A man, carrying a large camera case, was stood at a distance. When he glanced in her direction she felt herself momentarily drawn into some dark force field of panic. For a few seconds she was a four-year-old again, terrified of train stations and of being covered by the impending cloud of steam, soot and smoke – and she was also the little girl in the back of her parents' car, frightened by the story of the child murderer.

The feeling of panic and of being watched refused to go away. All during the holiday at her grandparents (who had stayed behind in the Midlands to free up their home) she was jittery – even insisting that her bemused husband drag the heavy television table across the bedroom door. She seemed to sense danger everywhere. On returning home the feeling subsided but left a trace of anxiety. It was though a window in her unconscious had been thrown wide open and then hastily closed – but in reality the window has been left slightly ajar. The young woman feels it takes a lot of her energy to pull on this window so that it won't blow open again in the slightest puff of wind.

The accommodation with the black be-speckled walls is an old coach house attached to the landlord's Victorian property, which is set in a pretty courtyard. During the summer months she'd placed a rickety chair by the front doorway (after choosing an LP from the minimal record collection comprised of 'The Moody Blues' and 'Iron Butterfly') and settled down to plan the future. The baby showed a preference for the heavy rock beat of 'Iron Butterfly' and merrily kicked away in the safety of an enclosed warm and watery world.

Throughout the autumn the young woman continues to reflect that she had done badly in her final term exams and was meant to be taking a year off to have the baby and think about the best way forward. Her mother's displaying an open-hearted attitude and has offered to help out if she decides to continue her studies. But the young woman thinks probably not – she wants to look after the baby herself.

The turn of the kaleidoscope is rapid. Despite studying hard her husband has no guarantee of employment after completing his degree and work placement. There is an atmosphere of discontent within the country as the miners plan to strike and an element of hardship pervades the lives of those struggling to care for their families on a minimum income.

Winter arrives and the house seems to absorb the cold and dampness on every level and no amount of rigorous scrubbing prevents the black mould from reappearing. The bedroom becomes untenable as rivulets of condensation run down the walls. But the bathroom is the worst affected. Friends refuse to use this room – they joke it has bad vibes like the scene of a murder. Once a week her husband lights the paraffin stove and she relaxes in a tub of warm bubble bath. The young woman's thoughts drift back to the memory of taking a bath as a child at her grandparents – when her grandfather would drag the large tin vessel (which hung in the back yard) in front of a roaring coal fire. He filled the pitted object from kettles heated on the kitchen stove – which was quite a feat considering he'd only one arm.

Now – in the murky bathroom, the warm water runs over the dome of her belly which gently undulates with the baby's kicking. The baby is a mystery in a lagoon of embryonic fluid. The young woman traces the shape of the infant's body, filling in details she longs to know. She tries to convince herself everything will come right – that in time her husband is bound to find permanent work and soon they'll be able to afford better accommodation. The baby is the brightest fragment in the shifting kaleidoscope pattern and with an effort of will it is possible to push all the darker pieces to the outer periphery.

Within this fractured landscape the young woman has no knowledge of Sun, Moon or Leopard. She is alone without their presence but there are books, words and thoughts. The books are plucked at random from the local library; Sartre, Plato, Galsworthy, D.H. Lawrence. The texts are a total hotchpotch of styles and ideas. There is no one to dictate to her what she should be reading, what she should be thinking.

But the questioning is always the same and the anxiety is always the same.

★ ★ ★

Leopard leaps back on the bed. 'I feel bad about this,' he says.

'Why?'

'I'm thinking I should have come to you sooner.'

'No need for that – I expect you were busy – giving guidance to someone in need. Remember – humans take a long time to reach a point of maturity – if at all, and I'm only part way through the story. But, shall I go on?'

'Yes – what happens next?'

The baby – a boy – is born in December. The unsuitability of their accommodation worries the young couple. They set up camp in the lounge downstairs where they eat, sleep and go about their daily lives. The rest of the house is abandoned to the biting cold and increasingly sodden walls. The young mother knows she must keep her spirits up – the baby boy is now the centre of her world and she owes it to this little person to do her best.

After a harsh winter of illness and various pressures the situation does improve. Spring follows – as it always must – and with one more turn of the kaleidoscope the young woman, her husband and their baby son move into their own home. Work is secure for the time being and an assured income means a few more LP's can be afforded. The little boy loves dancing to Neil Young's 'Till the Morning Comes'. He is just a toddler and does a little knee bend and bounce. Bounce, bounce – chuckle, chuckle – bounce, bounce – chuckle, chuckle – bounce, bounce – 'juice please mummy!'

The young mother, now twenty one, prefers grooving to John and Beverley Martin's 'Primrose Hill'. The carefree vibe evoked by the song doesn't quite fit with the reality of living in a terrace house situated next to a looming cement works but not to worry, she's only too relieved to have the luxury of a heated bathroom with its cheerful blue paisley wallpaper – and most important – not a spot of mould in sight. Now she can relax knowing that her toddler has an outdoor space to play in and a bedroom free from damp. The little boy has a white rabbit – Mr Nibs. The friendly creature hops around the enclosed garden following his playmate in expectation of sharing a packet of crisps. Watching the faithful animal and her son playing together warms the young mother's heart.

There is also an attic room – accessed by a shaky wooden ladder. With no extra money to furnish the space the young woman sits on a cushion and taps away on a second-hand typewriter. The inner questioning leaps into the typewriter keys and comes out as words. Poems and stories transform an underlying sense of anxiety into a medium that can be handled, fashioned and created into something meaningful. The young woman joins a local poetry group. She reads the poems with her new group of friends at pubs and cafés – it's a strange experience – this sense of finding her voice and the first small step of a very long journey.

The pieces of her life constantly rearrange. A pregnancy is sadly lost, but three years later there is another house move and then, soon after, the birth of a daughter. The young woman insists on a home birth – there is no way she is going through a repeat of a hospital delivery. She will never forget the unaccompanied journey in the back of an ambulance on a freezing December evening, prior to giving birth to her son. Husbands weren't allowed in the delivery room so she was packed off in the dead of night on her own. The labour was long and a group of student midwives gathered round her bed like a flock of squawking birds. One of the nurses had irritably tapped her fingers and told her to get a move on as she wanted to go for lunch. The afterbirth wasn't properly checked and three months later there was a repeat night-time journey in an ambulance because she was haemorrhaging. She remembers spending a week in hospital in emotional distress because the draconian rule of no visitation with babies or young children was still in place. To be apart from her little boy was unbearable and she had insisted on early discharge.

Three years later, the young woman has read about Leboyer's natural childbirth and is all prepared for a better experience, but things don't quite work out to plan. She goes into labour on the one night her familiar midwife is off duty. By early morning it's clear that something is wrong – the labour isn't progressing and she's in agony. At seven in the morning the relief midwife begins to panic and is soon shrieking down the phone at the regular midwife to come at once. All the young woman can hear are the words *face delivery* but she doesn't know what that means and is terrified her baby is going to die from oxygen starvation.

The midwife she knows and trusts is with her within minutes. The panicky midwife is sent on her way and as there's no time now for a caesarean things have to take their course. The baby girl's face is bruised black and blue from where the inexperienced midwife had prodded, thinking it was the crown of the head. Miraculously the baby is otherwise in one piece. The trusted midwife – the heroine of the day – explains that face deliveries are a rare occurrence and they must congratulate themselves on bringing the little girl safely into the world.

The maturing mother had begun to study with The Open University when pregnant, and just a few weeks after the birth she is well enough to cycle to her local seminar. Life feels good! She is thrilled to have both a son and a daughter and everything seems on track.

Two weeks later she wakes with a peculiar sensation. It doesn't matter that it's sunny outside, there's a horrible black cloud of foreboding above her head. She holds her baby girl close. The peculiar sensation has nothing to do with the baby – it's as though it's come out of thin air. The doctor insists on post-natal depression – the young mother isn't so sure but she willingly takes the pills. So many pills – uppers, downers, sleepers – some days she feels like she's walking on clouds when pushing the baby's pram. She feels cheated that these precious early months of her relationship with her baby daughter are passing in a blur.

The bemused young mother tries to think back to a familiar anxiety she'd experienced prior to the birth of her son. The low feeling had waxed and waned after the birth and eventually she'd agreed to medication – but the thing that had really helped was the writing and moving away from the mould-filled house. Is it the same low feeling this time – she's really not sure? The medics are upsetting her – they advise not to have any more babies because *this* will only get worse each time. But what is *this*? Nobody really talks with her about *what* she's feeling. There's a bit of her that feels her mind has cracked open and what she sees and feels is not in any way delusion – but a heightened sense of the fragility of life. It just makes the love she feels for her children all the more intense. If the pills are supposed to quieten her emotions they're categorically not working.

Two years later she flushes all the pills down the toilet – unaware of the dangers of suddenly stopping. There is a period of time when she feels cut adrift as her brain chemistry readjusts but this turns out to be a cathartic turning point. Whatever *this* is she knows she has to face it, come to understand and not be ruled by *it.* Another leg of the journey begins.

Six years and one Degree later, when the children are settled at school, the twenty-eight-year old gains a place at a bricks and mortar University to study for a further degree in Philosophy and Literature. She reckons she's earned the right to consider herself disciplined in this area of her life – academically it's taken ten years to finally get to where she'd wanted to be at the age of eighteen. It hasn't been plain sailing but she's grateful for the chances she's been given and happy with what she's achieved thus far – but there's still a long way to go in many aspects of her life. Sorting out where she's at academically is the least of her difficulties.

Soon after, in 1980, there's a final house move. The newly purchased house is broken down – a complete shambles – but it's the garden that beckons. The plot of land is a rural jungle of grassy overgrowth, weeds, blackberry bushes and wild roses. The young woman has never been a gardener but some elemental need draws her in. There is a tangle here to be nurtured and sorted – it may even be that part of the answer to the nagging 'big question' might be found within this landscape.

There are many twists and turns over the future years encompassing work and relationships. Somewhere along the way I left this young woman behind but remember her fondly now, with more kindness than I allowed at the time.

★ ★ ★

'It's a sunny day,' Leopard remarks, 'shall we continue the story outside? You know, it's hard to imagine the garden as a tangle but I'm sure I would have liked it. Just think of all that long grass – the perfect habitat for a leopard.'

'Yes – there was something free and relaxing about its being overgrown. Taming nature takes a lot of work. Stephen and Amy loved playing Star Wars in the brambles – I seem to remember Chewbacca hanging from one of the bushes.'

'Chewbacca?'

'Sorry – he's a character from the film. The kids collected these plastic replica figures and Chewbacca was one of their favourites.'

'Mm… I like the name.'

'Anyway – the kids were growing up and so was I. Seven years later, in 1987, I met Matthew while we were both training to be psychotherapists.'

'What made you go in that direction?'

'It was maybe inevitable. The human mind – human emotions – fascinated me. Being in therapy had helped me to work out what I needed at the level of relationships and career, in order to live a fulfilling life. If philosophy is the language of the mind – psychotherapy is the language of the heart and emotions. To stay in balance I needed to be bi-lingual.'

'Would you say I'm bi-lingual?'

'Most definitely; you translate Leopard speak into human speak – that's a rare skill.'

'But, this bi-lingual state you were reaching for – is it hard for humans to come by?'

'It can be – I still don't find it easy.'

'Why's that?'

'Well – with the heart and emotions a state of ease may be found, but the mind has a tendency to constantly stray from a point of equilibrium. Reflecting back on this seems to underline that the draw of philosophy could be said to appeal to a certain pernickety state of mind. Lurking under the guise of all that *thinking* lies the quivering of the mind's distrust of itself. In fact, philosophizing is often an activity of *over thinking*.'

Leopard's attention has shifted. He is taking a swipe at a bee hovering close to his nose.

I shoo the bee away and persist in trying to gain Leopard's attention. 'Despite all the thinking, it's only when my mind is quiet and at rest that I feel anywhere close to an answer. Perhaps the stillness, the quietness, is the paradoxical answer?'

Before Leopard can reply we are diverted by a yapping noise coming from the house.

'It's the bookcase,' Leopard sighs.

I can imagine the books jumping and jostling, demanding to be read. I feel uneasy. 'How can I trust my own experience, my own thoughts, without making some reverential, referential move? And how can I believe that everything required to survive the assault of 'the big question' is here in the silence, in the cradle of emptiness that is my garden?' I voice my anxiety out loud.

Leopard looks perplexed. 'How can your garden symbolise emptiness when you fill it with so much significance?' he challenges. But I sense he's half-teasing as he winks a moist eye.

'By empty, I mean devoid of external influence, external thought.' I explain.

Some of the texts on the bookcase are making a very loud noise.

'Intertextuality!' they jibe. 'You fool, how can you imagine your mind is empty, that your thoughts can escape being an adulterated mixture of everything you have taken in?'

'Yes, and I have taken in so much; intoxicated on a heady brew of learning,' I fretfully respond.

Leopard snorts. 'Do you have to be so *dramatic!*' he admonishes. 'Whatever's gone in can be sifted out again.'

'How?' I demand.

'Oh – you know – by employing reflection, intuition and reason,' Leopard continues, but I can see he is distracted.

The creature's ears twitch as he sits in a state of alertness.

His head swivels full circle. A familiar sound has stopped him in his tracks.

There is an echo in my garden; there is an echo in every peaceful space I have inhabited. It is the laughter of my spirit child playing.

'What is the point?' I gently reiterate

'What is the point of the question?' she giggles, bright eyed with self-confidence and impish audacity.

Now she is skipping in and out of the flowerbeds, singing, 'Butterflies and honeybees, rose-petal perfume, bright yellow buttercups and orange striped caterpillars tickling the palm of your hand.'

'What are you doing?' I ask with adult perspicacity.

'Oh nothing,' she laughs, caring little for my discernment, 'and everything,' she adds, skipping on her way.

FOURTEEN

Sun's Dilemma

It is the ninth year in the cage.

Leopard has become increasingly at home in his surroundings. I have put the coveted PhD aside and concentrate within this immediate space. The acceptance of situation has not been easily won. The external world, a place Leopard and I sometimes refer to as *the theatre of noise and expectations,* still beckons. We have met with self-proclaimed healers on our journey who promise 'a return' in exchange for belief, positive thought and, of course, money.

When we ran out of all three of the above essentials, Leopard and I decided to travel alone. This has not been to ignore collective knowledge but it is certainly to ignore the opinions of others. Sorting out knowledge from opinion is quite a task.

'Don't you think opinions are based on knowledge then?' Leopard quizzes.

'That's a tough one. I suppose I see opinion as dictatorial – marked by a lack of openness – in contrast to knowledge which is an expansive form of communication open to growth and change.'

Leopard nervously scratches. 'We've met a lot of dictators in the garb of angels, haven't we?'

'Yes. The worse have been those who dictate that a person is necessarily responsible for their illness or its continuation.'

Leopard gives a hard stare and continues mid-scratch. 'None of that really appeals as an explanation for why children get sick, or why positive-minded adults die of cancer and other degenerative illnesses, does it?'

Now – I'm also scratching. 'Illness happens, it's part of life. Healers and therapists who refuse to accept the fragility of our world, and all it contains, damage people with their opinions.'

Leopard paces round in circles in an attempt to relieve an increasing sense of agitation. He is part of the spirit world and fears the spirit world is often misrepresented. Then, he reminds me of a time when I lived outside of my white skin. From within Leopard's mind an image, snatched from a memory of the white man's colonisation of jungle, comes to the fore. We remember how the shaman was powerless in the force field of the white man's diseases, especially the flu viruses. The shaman watched his people die.

The shaman's people did not die of an unhealthy lifestyle, lack of positive thinking or the presence of negative entities, although the white man was a negative force. They died because their immune systems were not programmed to cope with foreign viruses.

We, who have so much knowledge, are required by destiny to inhabit two worlds and to learn two languages. We need to embrace the ancient spells close to our hearts and to reach for the overcoat of conventional medicine for additional warmth. Even leopards sometimes feel the cold.

'I expect thinking and expressing these thoughts takes a lot of energy,' Leopard observes.

'Yes – it does,' I acknowledge. 'That's why I don't speak in the human world very often.'

'Let's go into the garden,' Leopard suggests, knowing this will calm me.

'Words take so much energy,' I mutter. 'So much bloody energy!'

'Yes, sometimes they are red hot,' Leopard yawns, 'not white particles of light at all.'

Over many years Matthew and I have added to the landscape, plucking old buildings from their original owners. First we found a hut, complete with a roof tower and clock. The building was a former site office with a certain quaint charm. We spotted it in late summer when russian vine and honeysuckle cascaded above the door.

In late autumn the hut was dismantled by the original owner who seemed pleased with its potential home in our garden. The building had been the favourite haunt of his recently deceased mother. We christened the hut Trumpton (because of the clock) after the children's television programme. Trumpton arrived on a cold winter's day and Matthew and helpers worked in the snow to put the panels back together and tack on the roof. In the warmer weather Matthew painted the aluminium window frames and internal walls. The addition of bright sunflower curtains and rush matting completed our garden retreat.

The following year we recycled a timbered greenhouse. This time it was down to Matthew to dismantle and transport – a hard slog but worth it. In late summer, when the evening begins to chill, it's cosy to sit in the greenhouse with Sun streaming through the glass panes and the air pungent with the smell of tomato plants.

Last year Matthew created an additional pond by Trumpton, more formal than the wildlife pond. The water is clear and has become the home of frogs with Aztec markings.

This summer the nature pond resembles green pea soup and I spend the season trying to ameliorate the situation. The shelf in the summerhouse resembles an apothecary's lair with all kinds of potions for clearing the murky water and by late summer the meddling appears to have some positive effect.

It has been a strange summer. I hanker after even more space, more stillness – increasingly drawn towards the notion of living in a truly wild terrain, remote from man-made sounds. I am happiest when all that can be heard is the wind in the trees and birdsong, but even the birds can irritate. I am becoming more Leopard and less human and this is concerning.

Sun is also out of sorts. She languishes behind heavy cloud and angsts about a certain date and time (January 1st – 2000 – 3.59 am). Looking down upon Earth's bountiful estate she fixes her vision upon the Chatham Islands.

This tiny place is destined to be the first inhabited part of the world to witness Sun's rising at the start of the millennium. Sun wants to be seen at her most alluring. She dreams of a dress of orange hue, tinged with pink and scattered with thousands of pearly sequins.

Moon tells her not to worry, that humankind with their infernal technology will sort it. Moon stresses *infernal*.

'How will they sort it?' Sun asks, perplexed.

'Tethered balloons,' Moon smirks, 'high in the sky.'

Sun acknowledges this is a naff idea – she sniffs at the thought.

'Or, they might use strategically positioned cameras along the east coast of the islands,' Moon continues.

'But that means the show will be seen at sea level at a later point in time,' Sun wails, shifting her gaze through many degrees to the Balleny Islands, in Antarctica. Here Sun can pour her light for twenty-three hours a day, free to strut and play with dress. Here she is protected from the prying eyes of humans. Sun is caught between her desire for adulation and need of privacy. She hopes the humans won't come to the Balleny Islands with their cameras and clacking tongues. Her wish is that on the first day of the new millennium things in Antarctica will be as they have always been. Light on white, peace and calm – time experienced as nature's time.

FIFTEEN

I Spy With My Little Eye

Sun doesn't necessarily object to being watched. Her narcissistic streak delights in being sought after, admired and adored. If Sun could be sexed she would state that human adoration gives her a sublime, erotic thrill.

But some humans seek to deconstruct her. What started out as allure and mystery has been converted into an activity labelled 'scientific research'. Sun is embarrassed by the presence of peeping toms which now invade her personal space. The satellites wink and nod as they collect, collate and convey her innermost secrets to the earthlings below.

She shudders recollecting the sound of Ariane 5's engine, the fierceness of liquid oxygen and hydrogen being pumped into the ignition chamber by turbo pumps spinning at 33,500 RPM.

Sun had fizzed even hotter as the beast approached to observe her.

'What more do these earthlings need to know?' she'd

screamed at Moon, who felt a little jealous of her sister being the centre of attention.

The launcher eventually inexplicably veered off course, only reaching 13,000 feet before being blown up by the controller. The explosion represented a mere firework display to Sun, but Moon forcefully informed her naïve sister that tons of toxic chemicals had showered over the jungle of French Guiana.

'Where do you get all this information?' Sun asked.

'Oh – I just know about these things,' Moon replied, with an air of false modesty.

Meanwhile – Leopard puts his paws over his ears. He cannot contemplate the destruction of jungle.

Sun remains disconsolate. There is something distinctly intrusive, paranoia-inducing in being observed and monitored.

'What did they want to know this time?' she'd further enquired.

The reply tripped off Moon's tongue.

'Ariane was meant to launch a flotilla of four identical satellites intended to monitor in real time what humans call the solar wind.'

As a result of this information Sun is now constantly distraught. One of her favourite dances is so speedy she perspires – most profusely – and the minute beads of sweat form a stream of particles. The particles cascade to Earth, bashing and crashing into the planet's upper atmosphere causing, from time to time, the Northern and Southern lights.

'Why,' Sun demands, 'do humans need to know about such intimacies to appreciate my pyrotechnic show?'

'The trouble is,' Moon interjects, with a hint of spite, 'all that dancing does cause a bit of chaos.'

'How?'

'It's the sudden surges of power. You are responsible for shutting down televisions, navigational satellites and short-circuiting power grids.'

Sun pulls a face. 'Is that so very terrible?'

Moon remains complacent. She enjoys being in a superior position of knowledge considering she's had to take a back seat for aeons. Sometimes she thinks her sister is all brawn and no brains.

'You know this human commodity called money?' Moon minces, 'well, it's just that your antics cause a situation where a lot of money is used up.'

Sun feels a headache coming on. She longs for a past era, a time before she had to comprehend Cold War Politics and, more recently, the principles of multination partnerships aimed at dominance of a satellite launch market.

Moon senses her sister's agitation. 'The spending of money on research, they feel it's for the human good,' she offers, in more sympathetic mode.

'I do not understand this notion of human good!' Sun retorts. 'These humans are always askew. Remember the era of human sacrifice – I could have done without that! There is always some reminiscence of human stupidity to spoil the day.'

'I agree,' Moon concedes – casting a supportive glance in her sister's direction as she continues with her own evaluation of the situation. 'Perhaps the incineration of five hundred million pounds *is* a contemporary form of human sacrifice?'

SIXTEEN

Vertigo

The need for human sacrifice is possibly embedded in the human psyche. We may even feel something weirdly comforting in witnessing the pain of others. This isn't the sadism of a cruel heart but the attachment to a notion that there is possibly only so much bad energy to be dished out. We figure if some demonic god is to be appeased through human suffering perhaps we don't all have to endure in order to pay the bill.

We are free to sympathise, to let our compassion flow, as long as *that horrible thing* is not happening to us.

Some humans are so cut off from the possibility of becoming a victim of the worst possible circumstances they cannot even muster compassion. The twentieth century has become the receptacle of an amazing amount of theoretical garbage aimed at making the individual feel totally responsible for the vagaries of life.

A myth circulates that we can be omnipotent in regard to

health, work and relationships as long as we adhere to certain prescriptive ways of living.

Plain *bad luck* is ejected from the court of possible reasons for the harsh difficulties challenging some people's lives. Rejecting arbitrariness means we *always* have to come up with a reason. If we come up with enough reasons we inevitably have something to turn to, by way of protection or explanation. And there are so many protections to turn to.

'Don't you think it's natural to want to protect ourselves?' Leopard suggests.

'Sure, but what really angers me is having the opinions of others foisted upon me as a given.'

Leopard gives a playful growl. 'You still sound in a hot mood,' he teases, taking a swipe at the autumn leaves swirling down from the apple tree – and then continues, 'but you know your trouble?'

'I'm sure you're going to tell me,' I laugh, joining in the game.

'You get too strung out on your denials.'

'Don't you mean my rejections?'

'It doesn't matter what you call it,' Leopard explains. 'When we disagree with another's opinion we may be accused of denial or resistance, if the other person isn't open to the knowledge game. But I've tried to encourage you to analyse your denials, because resistance could be your intuition's way of informing you that a certain path is not correct for this present time.'

Leopard takes a flying leap into the air. 'Hey!' he roars, 'that was too many words. I'm getting as bad as you.'

Now he's dancing on hind legs. He makes four speedy

boxing movements with his front paws. 'Imagination (pow!) – curiosity (wham!) – openness (zing!) – reason (bam!) ... that's all you need to cope with a difficult issue.'

Leopard makes me laugh. I'm going to miss him when he's gone.

Meanwhile, I'm afraid of the arbitrary nature of life. Despite all the avenues of protection there are still particles of bad luck floating around out there.

For example, six weeks disappeared down a black hole at the beginning of the summer. It was early June and I'd been enjoying a better patch. After nine years of living with the same decor in the bedroom we decided to face the upheaval of decorating. The bedroom is my hermit's cave and the wall opposite the bed has been a changing landscape over the years. Once, it was filled with bookshelves until it finally dawned that facing all those books waiting to be read created negative energy. The shelves were removed and replaced by pictures and postcards with personal messages from friends.

I also painted a water scene – an attempt to visualise the illness and the potential for recovery – having decided that if I lived to my eighties it might be possible to steal back a few fragments of lost time. The watery landscape depicted many air bubbles meant to represent future years. Some of the bubbles were large and bright yellow, signifying special years hallmarked as the achievement of important goals. The picture was optimistic and though I don't know where it is now the belief in those energetic bubbles prevails.

The wallpaper, a splurge of blue splashed with impressionistic spring flowers had been up for years, predating my relationship with Matthew. The room was the last one in the house waiting to be redecorated and somehow it had become lost in time, along with its occupant.

But we got round to it. Down came the heavy green curtains to be replaced with shutters, recycled from slatted wardrobe doors. The stripped walls were painted a warm sunlight yellow. Dark spaces became light and fresh.

Three days later I woke with the world spinning, the bedroom having transformed into an inverted space which defied any attempt to position my feet on the floor (where was the floor?) Ever since childhood I've been afraid of throwing up – and given the option I'd rather walk on hot coals – so the intense nausea was also scary.

The inability to reach the phone induced an ominous sense of isolation. This is the sort of situation that triggers an inbred guilt/fear monitor, when I envisage every kind of worst scenario. I began to imagine what it must be like to be Matthew's mother living alone, despite being in her nineties. I am in the minds of the entire population of the elderly. Then I begin to think about worse illnesses than my own. What must it be like to have limbs that do not move at all, unable to attend to one's bodily functions? What about having a heart attack or stroke. Was I having a stroke?

Eventually, the spinning subsided and I stumbled my way to the sitting room and slumped into a chair – relieved to be able to sit half-upright. The garden felt still and calm in the early morning light and I sat quietly for a while, my eyes struggling to focus on the Philadelphus which was in full bloom. The white blossom exuded a sweet perfume and hung heavy with water droplets from the previous night's rain. Gradually my skewed senses began to disentangle, and – as hearing individuated from sight and smell – I sensed a slight humming in the air. Rising from my chair I shuffled across the floor to slide open the patio door.

The humming became more audible, a distinct sound singing over the ocean crashing in my ears. To an inextricably altered perception the sound echoed the cries of slaves incarcerated on a slave ship. I could visualize the bodies, smell the unwashed flesh and feel the distress. What once lay within the imagination had begun to leech into my senses. Yet I knew this subjective, unpleasant experience of vertigo was only a tiny fragment of the trauma of being tied to the deck of a slave ship.

I wonder if some human emotions are frozen in time, within the horror of their causal experience. Could it be that fragments of this frozen distress break free and float in a timeless space? And perhaps the fragments join together to produce a background noise – discernible to those who are also in distress but not to others who breeze through life. When we are forced to slow down (or choose to slow down) into the stillness, the silence, the noise is audible and our response is stronger than empathy.

Despair and courage, one sound mapped onto the other – this is a song of lamentation and also the dawn chorus – signalling what might be an intimation of hope or the start of another difficult day.

SEVENTEEN

The Guardian

The vertigo and nausea comes and goes but the ocean remains in my ears. It is more noticeable at night when the crashing of waves seems to mimic the heart's pounding. I have begun to get used to this new situation and tell myself I need no longer dream about moving near to the sea as it has taken up residence in my head.

Summer arrives, dragging its feet into August. Sun surveys her intimate solar calendar, a listing of dates predicting the ups and downs of her mercurial nature. Of late she feels low, distinctly out of sorts. She realises humans also experience mood cycles (just now expressed by pale faces and moans and groans) and hold her responsible for their 'lousy summer'. But Sun has a lot to contend with. Scrutinising the vast space defining her solar calendar she locates a star twinkling brightly next to a significant date – marked **December 1999**. It is the time designated by humans as her *solar maximum*.

Moon gleefully informs her sister *the Guardian* has been full of little stories about Sun's private life. Sun used to think *the Guardian* was a superior life form, an angelic presence ordained to divinely transmit important information to humans. Moon scathingly remarked that the title was merely that of a newspaper, a not all-together reliable method by which Earth's inhabitants attempt to disseminate information.

'So what does it say about me this time?' Sun enquires.

Moon scans Earth's surface and zones in on a human reading.

'It says that the solar maximum is the high point in an eleven year cycle. I'm afraid it all comes down to your causing chaos again.'

Sun feels herself blush, which will result in a warm day for humans.

'Why?' she asks tearfully, 'why is it going to cause chaos?'

'You suddenly heat Earth's atmosphere, and as it expands the satellites in low orbit unexpectedly slow down and fall.'

Sun is upset. She feels it is *she* who is about to fall. She is hotter than usual – disorientated and dizzy!

'I can't help it, it's all part of my natural cycle – they shouldn't put those stupid objects in my way!' she protests.

Earth is perceived as an annoying relative by Sun and Moon – a relative with irritating hangers-on known as humans or earthlings.

For once, Moon feels sorry for her sister. All this prying has begun to pass Moon by as she no longer perceives herself of any great interest. At first she was sad not to be the site of magical or fantastical stories; having disappointed the mythmakers with her barrenness, her uninhabited state.

Admittedly there is still some speculation – in a rather clinical way – but the imaginative element has waned. Yet Sun continues to fascinate and humans openly display their desire of her.

'I cannot always give them what they want, you know. There are forces beyond me,' Sun weeps.

Moon listens to her sister's frustration and is jolted into the recollection of a brief contact with the forces Sun refers to, though it was many aeons ago. She remembers a warmth in her being that gradually dissipated into the numbness of her freezing lunar nights. Moon recalls a story once told of the danger of Earth descending into the coldness she now endures. But Moon cannot recall any details of the story and it seems her sister has retained mere fragments.

What was the force behind the force?

EIGHTEEN

A Total Eclipse of the Sun

Whilst Sun is conscious of her role to play in the advent of the new millennium, Moon continues to keep a nervous tension under wraps. A reminder, gleaned from a previous year's oracle concerning her potential celebrity status, is etched upon her mind.

As darkest hour looms, Solar fans look West
The Guardian – August 8 – 1998

For a whole year, since reading the oracle, Moon has revelled in a state of excited anticipation concerning her role in this 'darkest hour' (when she will glide across her sister, causing a total solar eclipse). There hasn't been a total eclipse in mainland Britain for more than seventy years – little wonder Moon is excited at the opportunity to show off.

Moon surveys Earth's landscape and spies the West Country. She concedes within herself that at a global level her favourite dance is no rare event. This means she will have to rely upon a flurry of local interest to boost her self-esteem.

Yet Moon feels magical when she glides across Sun. This movement unsettles the normal way of things as petals tightly close and bird song ceases. Moon's dance causes dark shadows to flit across Earth's surface and humans momentarily feel in touch with the forces that used to be.

Leopard also dreams up a ritual as a vision unfolds within the space between his yellow-green eyes.

In August Leopard plans for us to leave the cage. He is building up stealth to cope with the event. We are to travel by Moon's light, joining the long line of pilgrims making their way to the West Country. We will not dwell upon the fact this pilgrimage is seen as a commercial challenge to those who want to 'promote Cornwall for pleasure and business'.

No, Leopard and I will shut out the tacky nature of twentieth century commercialism and focus our mind on shamanistic practice.

Moon plans to wear a sparkling yellow dress and she will shimmy whilst hurling a dark piece of fabric between herself and Sun. Yet the dance is only a mischievous spectacle and the darkness merely an interlude. The shadowy sky will not signify the darkness of emptiness and fear but the magical reversal of all that is familiar.

Leopard's Dream

Leopard watches the child run down to the water's edge. Her limbs move freely and she laughs with delight at this reclaimed pleasure.

Then, she glances up at the sky and admires Moon's new dress, made from a fabric of dusky grey – stitched with hundreds of glittering yellow stars. The fabric is gracefully draped over Moon's cratered bones.

The waves speak to the child. They tell her the light, which is present before Moon's dance, will disappear and become the past.

There is a rustling sound in the wind as the air chills, followed by an eerie silence. The landscape is mysteriously enveloped by darkness as Moon flings the black fabric screen before her sister. For a moment, a moment which feels like an eternity, the child is terrified. Spectral voices echo in her head, reminding her this is what it is like every time she gets sick. She is lost in the dark space and the misery feels eternal. It seems in those moments that time has become stuck – and as long as time goes on being stuck then nothing will pass. The dark space is trapped within the boundary of time and the natural, flowing nature of time paradoxically seems static.

The child senses Leopard's warm breath on the back of her neck. He whispers that to focus on time is to lose the significance of the space. To lose the significance of the space is to become a captive to a certain notion of time.

Moon sings, a steady rhythmical singing in synch with the intonation of an African drumbeat. Leopard rises on his hindquarters and snarls into the darkness. The child feels a *presence* as the events of her life – all of its joys and sorrows – rush past. She senses this awareness is an energy vibrating through the earth's core, an energy that can never truly disappear.

Leopard's paws pick up on the vibration as he pounds and splashes the water's edge. A surge of cosmic energy courses through his body and he begins to run – faster and faster – disappearing into the distance and darkness.

The child feels a pang of sadness. She realises Leopard is gone from her, that his healing powers are needed elsewhere. There is no fear because she trusts the creature will always re-appear in dreams. She might even learn to meet him in the jungle, which is his true home.

The crowds cheer as Moon makes one last pirouette and her sister is again revealed, wearing a vibrant, pearl strewn dress. The sisters give each other a coy, congratulatory smile – knowing they've put on a magnificent show.

The child looks up at Sun and calls out, 'Meet you in the back garden – no particular time but a very particular space.'

Interlude

Where is a good place to end a story when you're stepping in and out of a dream?

Maybe we made it to Cornwall – maybe not. Leopard and I may have simply got tired and decided to enter the long sleep.

But if you are reading this, one thing is certain. Our universe has survived into the Millennium, and Sun will no doubt be trying to seduce you away from words, and Moon will be continuing to strike an enigmatic pose at the time of New Moon.

This *constant* is our link between past, present and future – the only remaining fragment of a story we have long since forgotten.

PART TWO

2000 – 2014

NINETEEN

2002

Awake

I am still awake. The calendar has moved on a couple of years and I have neither the courage nor inclination to enter the long sleep.

The years are threaded through the eye of a needle in the belief that some value can be stitched from the past. I embroider clouds to hang above my bed, and uterine cavities containing tiny pearl beads held fast by silver threads – a safe haven for our future grandchildren. Over the past few months art has become a process of survival – a mode of expression and an adventure deep into the unconscious.

It never occurs that I have any ability for artistic expression until we buy a digital camera. The camera is a joint gift to each other in recompense for not being able to go on holiday. I start out safe by taking the usual snaps; flowers in the garden and still life on the kitchen table.

A few months later we arrive at a June day, a day marking the beginning of the summer solstice. I haven't thought about Sun for quite a while – not in an active way. Of course she's been loitering in the background, regarding me as a reluctant playmate because I've been out of sorts and ignoring her flirtations.

Leopard revisits the garden, as quietly and unexpectedly as he first arrived. *Stealthily* he would say. I catch a glimpse of him as he paces slowly across the lawn, eventually lying down at my feet. It strikes me he is no longer agile and sleek. Leopard omits to explain where he's been the past two years but merely continues the conversation we've always shared.

'Did you really think it was going to be that easy?'

'Easy?'

'You know – to stay positive, to make something good come out of a difficult situation?'

'No,' I reply, hugging him, 'but I didn't think it would be as challenging as mastering alchemy!'

'I'm glad you've returned,' I confide, the tears welling up. 'I have failed to stay positive – I'm often angry and complaining. Why can't I hold onto the space you showed me?'

Leopard gazes at me and behind his misted eyes I sense compassion.

'So – things haven't been too brilliant?' he asks, settling down on his haunches.

'No – it's been challenging! I should not have sent you away.'

'Hmmm … I don't recall that you actually sent me away?'

'Perhaps not directly, but I wanted closure with a neat yet

slightly enigmatic ending. I left you running along the beach – in the opposite direction to the one I was headed for.'

'You thought you could leave part of yourself behind?'

'Are you part of me?'

'Surely,' he replies, rolling onto his back and closing his eyes against Sun's rays in a gesture I remember well, 'but this is something you have always known.'

'Don't go to sleep Leopard,' I urge, there are things I need to tell you.'

'Oh – can I listen too?' a small voice pipes up. The child is back, sitting amongst the branches at the base of the apple tree.

The June heat is soporific and there is a shimmering in the air, creating the visual effect of placing Leopard and the child behind an opaque veil. I squint in an effort to focus.

'Leopard – I have this new camera – it's brought a bit of magic into my life.'

'Magic … are we going to talk about magic?' the child gasps and claps her hands, 'that sounds fun!'

'Do you know – with a few scraps of crepe paper, a torch and some silver foil you can photograph a galaxy?'

'What – you just point the camera, press a button and hey presto?' she laughs, jumping down from the tree.

Leopard gives a loud snort.

'Ok – it's not quite that simple. I have to put the image on the computer and then I do a bit of colour mixing and maybe some blending – but it's just like painting.'

'But you don't get paint everywhere,' the child smiles, 'probably not messy enough for me.'

'I'd like to take some self-portraits but I seem to have a

bit of a block,' I persevere, trying to get Leopard's attention but the snort is now becoming a snore.

'Leopard, please try and stay awake while I tell you this because it's bugging me.'

'Oh I know all about the problem,' the child butts in. 'Lie down and have a little snooze and the story will come back to you in a dream?'

'It will?'

'Oh yes – and when you wake up you'll know exactly what to do.'

★ ★ ★

THE SELF PORTRAIT

The eleven year old is settling in at her new school and thinks her mother will be pleased with the term's report which says she is making *'encouraging progress'*. Her form teacher is a sweet natured elderly woman – not fierce like some of her colleagues. Along with the rest of the class the child is in love with their young French teacher who is sadly leaving to have a baby. The teacher promises the girls she will bring the new baby in for them to see.

All in all things are going well. Admittedly maths is a foreign land the child struggles to familiarize herself with but the eccentric maths teacher, who looks a bit like Einstein, has taken a shine to her. In future years she will become the teacher's babysitter and spend many happy hours looking after his second family of two baby girls, the widower having re-embarked on marriage and fatherhood in his sixties.

The only damp squib on the report is the comment of her art teacher. He has simply scribbled *fair.*

The art teacher is a young man with a smooth aquiline countenance which contorts into a nervous smile when trying to deal with the high spirits of his pupils. In her adult life, the child will come to recognise this awkward manner as the consequence of a boarding school education. The class atmosphere is a strange mix of the vibes given off by the girls, who love to push the boundaries, and the jittery gestures of a staff member who is clearly out of his comfort zone. For his pains the young man must also double as a music teacher. Every music lesson descends into chaos as the girls deliberately warble and sing off key.

But the class get their come-uppance. The child is prepared for the usual splash around with paint during the art lesson – and hopes that she and her new best friend might be chosen as paint monitors whose task it is to stay behind and generally tidy up. For the young girls this is seen as an opportunity to try and engage the young man in conversation – the truth is, in comparison to most of the male teachers, his whimsical nature is quite good fun.

Lisa and the child are still friends but they have spread their wings. Lisa has chosen the prettiest girl in class to be her special friend but the child doesn't mind as her own new best friend has a sensible and down to earth personality, whilst still being fun, and they seem to be a good match. She has been to the new friend's house for tea and notes the atmosphere is more relaxed than at home. Her friend's mother is cheerful and confident and loves to chat while they all sit round the table and eat what she calls her 'thrifty dinners'. If there's tension in the house (her friend insists that her younger siblings can be annoying) it doesn't seem to bubble over as things are apt to do at home.

This day the art teacher hands out a single piece of drawing paper and a piece of charcoal. The young man clears his throat before giving out instructions. 'Now girls, I thought it would be good for you to draw a self-portrait and you can take it in turns to introduce yourselves and say a little bit about how you're settling in at school.'

The child immediately feels sick. 'Please, please don't let me get a lump in my throat!' she chastises within herself – picking up the piece of charcoal under the pretence of making a start because some of her classmates are already confidently drawing.

She just knows her picture is going to be awful – that the self-portrait won't look anything like her true self. Putting down her piece of charcoal she judges the drawing as silly and childish. The picture is a pathetic round circle with scrawling for hair – and the eyes, nose and mouth are all in the wrong position.

Then – horror of horrors! The class monitor is instructed to gather all the work and take it to the teacher's desk. This is worse than the original plan. A guessing game is put in operation as the teacher holds each picture aloft and with his whimsical smile – that no longer looks quite so endearing – demands, 'and who do we think this is?'

It's not as though the child's picture is the only one to be laughed at. There are just two drawings in the entire pile that stir admiration for their evident artistic talent.

But the child feels a real sense of shame. She is hot and

sticky, blushing from head to toe as she is forced to walk to the front of the class to collect the travesty of a piece of art.

Art is dropped for domestic science at the first opportunity and is not seriously thought about for the next forty years.

TWENTY

Multiplication

'There are more newts in the pond than ever before,' Leopard remarks.

'Yes – that's the second thing I wanted to tell you about but just let me clear my head from sleep.'

It is true – clearing the pond of weed has become a newt-spotting game. The creatures cleverly embed in the green mass, some as tiny as the end of my little fingernail. I gently tease the silvery bodies from the green matting, anticipating the tickling sensation as they wriggle on the palm of my hand. The bigger newts have attitude. They emerge from the weed on their own steam and look me in the eye as though to say, 'Hey, I was having a nice sleep, did you have to disturb me?' Then, they sliver across my palm and dive back into the water. They are graceful swimmers.

'Did you notice,' I say, with a hint of pride, 'all of the ponds have water lilies now?'

'Mmmm … I saw you sitting by the edge of the big pond

dangling your feet in the water. What were you thinking about?'

'A lake in France; I was trying to submerge one of the water lilies in the pond and my toes became wrapped in the leaves. It reminded me of swimming across the lake.'

'Did that make you sad?'

'Only for a moment; I'm lucky to be able to create a garden that brings to life so many memories.'

'The garden has grown, it has changed,' Leopard observes.

'How can the same space grow?' a small voice interrupts.

'Ah – I see you are still with us,' I acknowledge, 'thank you for the dream – very illuminating.'

'Well it was your dream,' the child replies – raising an eyebrow. 'But how?' she demands, 'How do you make the space bigger?'

I often think about this conundrum because the garden does seem larger. The old rubbish tip at the very end of the plot is now a wildlife space. We eventually added another pond and planted large structural plants. The birds hide beneath the elephant ears and the bees feast on the flowers the plants produce. In May, a carpet of bluebells covers the area. The flowers exude a smell redolent of springtime walks with my father. As the bluebells die down, tissue-layered poppies, lush ferns, hostas, rosemary and alliums, replace them. The earth has a rich, onion smell; the aroma of my grandfather's allotment. In an instant I am a child again, running down the lane ahead of my grandfather; careful to avoid any foraging hens because they terrify me with their clucking and flapping.

Sometimes I think the garden is too stuffed and it is like

when my mind feels too full of words. Then I have to clear spaces, allowing things to breathe. When my mind needs clearing I go into the garden and sit quietly. I've become re-accustomed to the bird song – it no longer troubles me. I listen to the wind and the bird song and become calm.

The child tugs at my skirt. 'How,' she demands, 'how do you make the space bigger?'

'You make the space bigger by increasing the metonymic chain,' I reply.

'What on earth does that mean?' She has a look of exasperation.

'It means giving symbolic meaning to everything in the garden. All the plants and animals get tangled up in a web of meaning and memory.'

The child seems uncertain. She walks over to a flowerbed and points to a snapdragon. 'What does that mean?'

'It reminds me of when I used to be you. I was mesmerised the first time dad pinched the petals to make them open and close like the mouth of a dragon. Here, let me show you.'

I pinch the petals on a fiery red plant. The child giggles but when I turn round she is gone.

'Does she still do that?' Leopard enquires

'You mean disappear? Yes … she does it all the time,' I frown. 'I can never find her.'

TWENTY ONE

2003
A New Direction

The beauty of digital photography is that I can work on the images from my bed. The computer has become an art studio, with every paint pot and brush available at the click of a mouse.

All of the images are photographed on the kitchen table and it's quite an arbitrary affair. I can never be sure what will result from this mixing of luminosity – created with torch or lamplight shone upon crepe papers, silver foil and hessian. The serendipity of whatever emerges from the process of downloading images to the computer screen is exciting.

During the past year I've put together a portfolio and have decided to put on a solo exhibition. Matthew is now proficient at mounting and framing the art work which has been printed off on our new A3 printer. We are learning a range of skills at a rate of knots.

Sun and Moon are curious.

'What does it say on the poster?' Sun enquires.

'It says *image and imagination*. I don't mean to boast but there's a beautiful picture of me above the title!'

Sun attempts to quell her jealousy. 'Well – I saw all the pictures for the exhibition the other day and there are loads of me.'

'But they're not really *of* us are they – we're just the inspiration,' Moon interjects. She senses an argument is brewing. The trouble is her sister gets on her nerves and it's hard to hold back.

Sun isn't about to let things go. 'I happen to think it's very important that we're a source of inspiration to the humans. There would be no poets or artists without us.'

'That's true,' Moon concedes – but thinks to herself that the lunar images are the most arresting. The photographs are luminescent and evocative – but best of all she is portrayed in a series of dresses to die for. She is clothed in blues, pinks, turquoise and white. Her favourite image is one in which she's depicted wearing a garment made from white silk – edged in purple.

The fashion show element isn't lost on Sun. She sees herself rising, floating, and sinking within ethereal landscapes – and to her delight she is captured wearing a dazzling array of dresses. Her favourite is a blood-red shift dress set off beautifully against an indigo blue mountain, behind which flashes of yellow and green light erupt like flames across a golden sky.

Moon finds some of the more sombre images disquieting. There is one in particular where a ghostly apparition of a white bird (or is it a trick of light against a lunar skyline) swoops above her cratered body. The bird seems to encompass all of space and Moon senses that a sensitive human may become lost in the image – may shelter under the white bird's wing and for a little while rest in a state of peace.

TWENTY TWO

Another Report Card

The most unnerving aspect to the exhibition is the fact I fail to mentally prepare for a 'comments book'.

'I didn't realise,' I explain to Leopard, 'that the gallery keeps a book and give me a photocopy of all the comments. What if people think my work is crap – what if everybody just writes *fair?*'

Leopard guffaws, 'and what if people think it's great? Knowing you – you'll struggle with that as well!'

Let's just say the ensuing positive affirmation is heart-warming and encouraging. Sun and Moon are far more puffed up than me – they think the exhibition is all about *them,* which in some respects is true.

The exhibition unexpectedly acts with the force of an erasure over the past. I nervously scan the 'report card' which is to be held in perpetuity by the gallery. Just as with all those prior school assessments, from long ago, it functions in the present as a written commentary on my ability and the part of me lacking in confidence expects to read failure.

The feedback that seems to matter most is from my family – who all attend the exhibition. I hadn't really expected my parents to visit the gallery, thinking it would evoke in my father the same anxiety that resulted in the missed open evenings when I was a child.

My mother has written in her beautiful, neat handwriting,

Well done, much deep thought given. Excellent exhibition.

All of the doubts embedded in my mind are rubbed out and written over with those few words.

It's funny how the past can hit us like a tsunami, reduce us to tears and then carry us to a further shore where we feel strangely healed.

TWENTY THREE

Let's play Dressing Up

The eleven-year-old had struggled to produce an image resembling the self she recognised in the mirror – would the fifty-year-old have the same struggle? This is what I ponder as I prepare for my first photo-session of self-portraiture.

What is a *real self* anyway – especially when we remove our physicality? Is it the thoughts and feeling we express to others – is it all the thoughts and feelings we wouldn't dream of expressing? Is it an amalgam of the two?

I ransack the wardrobe and an old suitcase, ending up with an odd assortment of dresses and costumes.

Costume One – the pink ballet tutu.

Eyes stare straight at the camera lens. What do these eyes want to say? I think they say I am still a dancer in my heart – this photo is my defiance. I light a cigarette but it's only a prop – I haven't smoked since my twenties. And even then a cigarette was just a prop – a smoke and a glass of whisky – the closest I would ever come to dependency on mind altering substances.

'Really …what about the pills?' Leopard interjects.

'The pills? Yes – I'd forgotten about those – addiction courtesy of the NHS.'

Audition for Dallas.

I feel guilty about this costume – an antique dress with a long, flowing red skirt and low cut strapless bodice. It belonged to a friend a long time ago and I was meant to return it.

I'd also borrowed a creation made from pink silk. My daughter wore it for her tenth birthday party dressed up as a Victorian beauty – her long blond hair curled tight and a string of pearls about her neck. I still have the photo and she is loveliness personified and then static loveliness is healthily trashed in another photo of the young friends racing up the garden to hang out in the old apple tree – party dresses hitched up to the waist and curls blown free in the wind.

The red dress is from another time – another life.

The first photo I take is glam – Matthew really likes it and runs off a copy to frame. It is given the title 'Audition for Dallas'. But the second photo is more authentic – it is sad and pensive. I give it the title *Waiting.*

Taking the photos is proving exhausting. I have to keep resetting the delay timer on the camera and repeatedly walking across the room is causing my calf muscles to fill with lactic acid. Tomorrow's going to be a rough day, but I'm having fun and it's hard to stop.

Next I try out a series of outfits and hats. The hats once belonged to Matthew's mother and I title this series *Grandma's Hats*. I am very fond of my mother-in-law who has always been kind to me despite being a tough old bird. I admire her resilience in working through to her seventies running a market stall and in her nineties she is still mentally sharp and likes to discuss politics. I wish I could spend more time with her but the geographical distance makes it hard.

I can't fasten the buttons on my wedding dress (which matches a cream hat) and conclude I must have been ridiculously thin when Matthew and I got married. I wonder what I can do with the dress and think it would make a nice christening gown.

In the end only a few of the photos are of any interest – but a part of me has fallen in love with the camera – with this activity.

'It's got nothing to do with narcissism,' I say to Leopard.

He almost explodes with one of his derisory snorts.

'Ok – maybe just a little bit. You have to admit that glam photo looks pretty cool. But the ones I really like are when there's no discernible difference between what lies behind the eyes – the emotions behind the gaze – and what the camera captures as a static image. It's like the camera lens has gone deep inside my thoughts and there's no place to hide – I simply have to give it all up and not be afraid to share. I'm going to repeat those ballet pictures every decade.'

'Er … I don't think you're going to be fitting into that tutu in ten years' time,' Leopard candidly remarks.

'Probably not – I'll just have to buy another one!'

TWENTY FOUR

2005
Echoes

I still experience the crashing of waves in my ear. When the crashing subsides it leaves an echo, akin to the trace of a high-pitched wail. The wailing travels on the wind, sweeps under the gaps of doorways and squeezes through the cracks and crevices of walls. My ear is an echo chamber – reverberating with the sound of the misfortune of others in advance of the global news machine.

AS A NEW YEAR DAWNS, THE WORLD REMEMBERS THE
TSUNAMI DEAD.
The Guardian – January 1st – 2005

To remember? 'What does it mean to remember?' I ask Leopard.

It is a cold, grey day and he is curled up at the end of the bed. He slowly lifts his head and pensively stares at me. Far more ill than usual – I have lived within this gaze for the past seven weeks.

I can't be sure what precipitated this severe relapse – possibly the combination of working towards another exhibition in the autumn of 2004, along with other projects. The illness has a dominant will of its own and often hits back hard if I don't meekly follow.

The bed is hemmed in by a commode: a Zimmer: a food trolley and numerous plastic boxes containing essentials. The desk has become a galley kitchen and the conservatory additional lying-down space. Most days I'm unable to walk the dozen steps from the bed to this additional space.

'What does it mean to remember?' I reiterate.

'Perhaps what you're really asking is what is it to be remembered?' Leopard suggests.

Leopard always manages to turn words round so I can never ask a simple question.

'How do we remember the dead with whom we have no personal, immediate connection?' I continue in exasperation. 'Today's memory of the tsunami victims rises from the ashes of our memory of the victims of Darfur, the victims of the Palestinian conflict, the shadow of the Twin Towers. The list is endless. We do not retain this list in our minds but it becomes part of our collective unconscious. We pride ourselves on understanding the nature of shared responsibility as we dig deep into our pockets and give generously.'

Leopard yawns. Ignoring him I continue to ramble on.

'A second later we flip through the travel supplements of the Sunday newspapers and are informed that the best place to chill out for the New Year is South America. There are so many exotic places to visit – so many interesting and expensive ways to *lose* our hearts.'

I stop for a minute to catch my breath before rattling on. 'Don't fancy travel, then get yourself down to Harvey Nichols, Selfridges, and Debenhams for a spot of retail therapy. We are encouraged to remember and we are encouraged to forget. Forgetting wins hands down every time.'

'You are on a rant,' Leopard sighs, 'why bother with the newspaper if it aggravates you?'

'Because I'm afraid if I can't hear this clamour of voices I might as well not be here!'

Leopard wrinkles his nose in a gesture of disdain.

'You've been lying in this room for the best part of fifteen years; surely you've worked out it's only the clamour of egos you can hear?'

'I know that Leopard, but every now and then you hear a genuine voice.'

I have been ruminating recently because it is winter both outside and inside my room. Being confined to bed, and too unwell to keep up a meaningful connection with the external world, has precipitated a downward spiral into low spirits.

In the summer, before this latest relapse, Matthew inherited a tiny bungalow near the sea. We are grateful to an aunt who thought on a gift of future security for Matthew when he was a small boy. With no children of her own, her nephew brought purpose and happiness to her life.

Decades later, the once small boy – who spent every summer of his childhood playing on a beach with his aunt – is now approaching pensionable age. The spectre of aging is stalking us, poking us between the shoulder blades. How can it be, were we not young when all *this* began? I should have been working all these years, building up my little pot of gold – coins for the children, coins for the grandchildren, coins for the medical bills, coins for the eventual incarceration in some godforsaken care home.

The bungalow (which backs onto a field and an ancient wood) beckons – a place of rest in a chaotic world. I love to watch the seagulls from the bedroom window as they swoop down upon the newly ploughed field. In the distance they appear as freshly fallen snow.

But travel is out of the question as a mere trip to the bathroom induces dizziness, the world spinning – just as it really does – on its tilted axis.

The thought of our retreat tugs at my mind – a tantalizing memory amidst the bleakness of the present situation. A photo of Sun (taken the previous spring) hangs on the wall opposite my bed at home. The photo captures her rising over the fields. I had woken early that morning to be greeted by Sun wearing her best party frock ever.

'See', she beckoned, 'it's all gossamer.'

The gossamer floated in misty layers across the horizon – the fabric undulating and tangling within the branches of an ancient oak tree. The tree stands rooted – a guardian of nature's time – in the far corner of the field.

'Come on,' Sun shrieked, 'I can't stay dressed like this forever!'

'But,' I protested, pointing at my dowdy bathrobe and slippers, 'I'm not dressed for a party.'

'Rubbish!' she admonished. So still in bathrobe and

slippers, grasping my camera, I stumbled into the garden to record her celebration attire.

The image hung on the bedroom wall for three years – until I was able to make the journey once again.

TWENTY FIVE

Heartbreak

How many times can a heart break?

We learn to recognise a familiar ache or twinge which acts as a cautionary reminder that strings are being pulled taut – strings deftly attached to the past.

My father came by himself to the autumn exhibition of 2004. The images were entitled 'Painting on Snow'. Earlier in the year there had been a spectacular late snowfall as blossom and spring flowers disappeared beneath a white canvas. With great excitement I mixed some watercolours to see what effect could be achieved by painting on snow. I thought maybe this had been done many times before but I'd never seen a snow painting and wondered if the process would work.

The watercolours bled into the snowflakes which continued to softly tumble down. I retrieved an old tin tray and spatula from a kitchen cupboard and proceeded to scoop, and then compress the flakes into the tray. I had to work fast because the snow melted rapidly when brought indoors. The result was a series of photographed images that became the basis for the exhibition.

As always, Sun and Moon perceived themselves as models draped in a new season's collection of dresses. On this occasion the luminosity was created by the sparkle and glitz of tiny ice crystals.

'Cor! Wow! I look like a huge glitter ball hung in the sky,' Sun exclaimed.

'Well – I think it might be said that I look a little mysterious,' Moon coyly suggested – she really wished her sister wasn't so common at times!

I had not expected to see my father when we went for a final look at the exhibition. It was late afternoon and dad was a lone figure in the gallery as he stood, bent over – gazing intently at one of the pictures. I felt an ache in my chest – over my heart – wondering what he was thinking and waited quietly by the door as he went round the gallery spending time with each picture.

Despite sometimes making fun of himself my father is an emotional, sensitive man. He initially struggled to accept my health had been felled in one swift swoop and in the early months stood at the end of the bed nervously suggesting a brisk walk in the fresh air would surely do the trick. This only resulted in my tetchy response that as there was no pleasure to be had in my lying immobilized week after week surely it was obvious I'd go for a walk if I could?

In these latter years he is apologetic concerning his initial reaction and often visibly upset by the loss of my health, my work and its value to others. His recognition seems to have released me from an innate fear that I'd positioned myself outside of the family fold – too full of self-belief, too arrogant – too puffed up with my 'fancy education'.

Sadly, my father infrequently visits on his own so I'm rarely able to have the conversations with him I'd like but sometimes the communication comes in other ways – a book left on the doorstep with a little note, a bundle of plants for us to put in the garden and the frequent assurance that on his regular visits to mass I am in his prayers. For many years now my parents have had a 'truce' and follow their respective religious traditions.

I often worry that my family feel excluded by my illness and try to understand how this situation must impact from their point of view.

This is a subject Leopard and I frequently return to – the problem of how to negotiate so many different points of view.

A point of view is the wellspring of all the stories we create about others and our own lives. We swim in a sea of thoughts and opinions but who can say where the truth lies? *Truth* is a very tricky notion indeed.

Our chance meeting with my father at the exhibition was brief but afterwards I noticed a comment in the gallery book – written in his delicate handwriting composed of tiny letters adorned with flowing loops.

'Very appropriate on this 1st day of winter. Paula has captured the beauty we can look forward to.
Signed: *(DAD)*

How many times can a heart break? There was something concerning about my father's demeanour that day. I have always worried about him – from as far back as I can remember – but in 2003 he suffered a breakdown, probably caused by vascular dementia which unbeknown to us was silently inflicting great damage upon his mind.

In childhood we pick up on fragments of knowledge concerning our parents. To begin with it may be a certain look or a sudden outburst of temper or tears. As we grow we start to notice little idiosyncrasies – an attachment to certain items, tantrums if an object goes missing and stubbornness in the face of reason – all the forms of behaviour *we* are chastised for. We begin to learn that adults are children in disguise.

Growing up, it was easier to read my mother from these cues but my father's affable nature hid any complexity.

On reflection we can usually identify a cross over point (which is filled with tension) when our greatest desire as a child was to be a grown-up – whilst the grown-up we felt closest to simply wanted to be a child again.

Leopard sits pondering – sometimes he can't escape my silent, inner thoughts and comes in on what might seem like a tangent.

'I can remember you saying that humans take a long time to mature – is that because it's not so nice being a grown up? I can remember the fun I had when I was a cub – playing around in the long grass – it was exciting!'

'Sort of – I have another story connected to growing up – if you've time?'

'Time! What a strange thing to ask – remember, this room is a timeless zone.'

The child thinks she is very lucky because her father has a car and when the weather is fine they go out every Sunday afternoon for a picnic.

'We're going to the woods today,' she tells Lisa.

'Well – don't come back with some tale about seeing pixies and things 'cos I won't believe you!'

The child sighs; it is the time of year when the woods are full of bluebells and primroses and more importantly *magic*. She is certain her father believes in the magic – wasn't that the reason they visited the woods in spring?

Their mother seldom wants to come on walks – she is happy to stay in the car with her knitting and wave as her two girls run up the hill to the woods and disappear out of sight. But her father is in his element striding out and breathing in the sweet, spring air – occasionally stopping to shovel some leaf mould into a bag or pick dandelions for the pet rabbit and guinea pigs at home.

The child is excited thinking about how they will explore deeper and deeper until chancing upon a fairy grove. She and her big sister will tip-toe round a circle of toadstools, and peer into the cavernous space of a felled hollowed tree trunk that is now covered in soft green moss.

This is how it always is when they go to the woods.

★ ★ ★

Oh – to stay in that sacred, magical space forever!

I revisited the same wood as an adult but couldn't find the

exact spot – perhaps I even walked through it without realising. The disappointment was almost too much to bear. The magic grove is a place in my memory – a very special place – it is the place I loved my father most. In temporal reality it is lost forever.

As a small child I thought my father was the key holder to the magic – I didn't realise that I – the child – was the key that enabled him to escape his adult world.

Once a child knows this nothing is ever the same again.

★ ★ ★

A while later, the twelve-year-old – who is longing to be a teenager – feels that *knowing things* is a mixed blessing – especially as adults seem to think it's fine for children to know just half a thing.

Today is an important event – at least that's how she and Lisa see it. They have walked into town and are daring to buy a new item of clothing on their own.

'Well – which size do you think Lisa? I don't know how to work it out.'

'I dunno – what size is your jumper?' Lisa replies, roughly pulling at the back of her friend's neck to find the label. 'It says small – but that doesn't help. I think mum said I'm a thirty inch chest. What does it say on the packet?'

'I don't understand Lisa, it doesn't say chest – it says *bust* and look, it's got letters of the alphabet on it – this one says cup size B?'

Lisa snatches the offending package from her friend, laughing. 'Doesn't your mum tell you anything – it depends – you know – on how big you are?'

The young girl willingly goes with her friend's greater knowledge. It had been the same when discussing starting their periods. 'No-way-never,' was Lisa going to use, 'horrible! Old-fashioned! Dr Whites!' Lisa's mum had a neat little package of Libra pads ready for her in the airing cupboard.

'I'm not wearing some stupid girdle thing and then a cotton sausage with loops!' Lisa shrieked, with that mischievous arch of the eyebrow that had her admiring friend in fits of giggles. The young girl's mother had agreed to comply with this new modern method and handed over a booklet at the same time.

'This will give you the information you need dear – I expect I can leave it to the school to explain all that kind of thing.'

The school! The young girl thinks her mother is deluded – what could a witches' coven have to tell her about 'all that kind of thing?' You even had to *burn* the blooming things at school. It was so embarrassing – the stench from the incinerator – so the entire class was bound to know when it was your time of the month!

Never mind – Lisa was a fount of information – she and her group of friends could work it all out between themselves.

'I think I'm a small size Lisa,' the young girl deduces – thinking back to the furtive glances in the girls' showers after games lesson. No one wanted to get left behind in the growing up stakes and comparisons were frequently made.

'Here's a size A,' Lisa instructs, handing two packets over, 'do you want the one with the rosebuds or the plain white. *I'm* going to need a B.'

'The rosebuds – can't wait to try it on.'

At home, the young girl wears her new purchase for the rest of the day with a small vest, so that the outline of the bra can be seen and a small sliver of material with the rosebud pattern. She feels so grown-up and flounces from room to room hoping her father will notice. Eventually her mother prompts with a direct hint. 'Well – you'll never guess what's been bought with this Saturday's pocket money!'

'Oh – yes – very pretty,' her father grins as he makes a pot of tea in the kitchen, and goes whistling on his way.

The twelve-year-old sometimes thinks her father smiles his way through everything – it's his default position outside of the odd reactive outburst of annoyance. He's the sun coming out after stormy weather. To cause her father upset is painful and she's long concluded he's not as tough as her mother. It's a subtle thing and growing up she's observed that her father's been lined up in the defence regiment – whilst her mother is on some other side trained to initiate attack. There is something the young girl doesn't understand regarding adult relationships and the way in which her parents determine their respective positions. She hates being in the middle – never sure whose side to take but invariably runs to her father's defence. This just causes more stormy weather.

★ ★ ★

A little while after the shopping expedition the young girl has a premonition that the approaching summer holiday will be different. Things are changing within her family. They have moved into temporary accommodation, a smaller house on the estate whilst her parents have saved the deposit for their own home. Soon they will be moving into a nice semi-detached house, backing onto fields.

Her mother has already succeeded in nearly burning down the present house by leaving an electric fire too close to the clothes horse and now she has had an accident on her bike and dislocated her shoulder. There is some kind of mischief at work.

The temporary accommodation is opposite a playing field with a brook. The playing field has always been called the 'humpty dumpty' field because it undulates and the child and her friends played here when younger, rolling down the humps and then jumping up with glee at still being in one piece. The brook is shallow enough to paddle in with wellies and has tiny fishes. A steep pathway lays the far side of the brook and leads up to the House on the Hill. The building's tall spire dominates the skyline and can be easily viewed from a bedroom window. But play is not what it used to be. Lisa has also moved some way off to a newly built house and the group of friends who used to hang out in the street and 'the bushes' has dispersed. Her older sister spends a lot of time at her boyfriend's and won't be coming on holiday with them this year.

Somehow, the young girl feels the thought of going to her grandparents isn't so exciting. If it wasn't for her little sister there would be no enthusiasm for the packing of buckets and spades and favourite summer dresses. But her little sister is excited and this is infectious.

'Will there be donkeys?' the three-year-old asks.

'Oh yes – and we can go to the fair. It's huge you know –

with loads of rides and there are candyfloss stalls and if you're good dad might buy you a toffee apple.'

Listening to the sound of her own voice is giving the young girl a strange feeling in her tummy – she can hear herself talking but it's like she's a bit removed. This is a new experience. She is telling her little sister a story about going on holiday but she's not really *feeling* it. There's another peculiar thing keeps happening – sometimes when she looks in the mirror she doesn't quite recognise herself. She blinks hard and hopes the funny feeling will go away.

Week one of the holiday and it will soon be the young girl's thirteenth birthday. She hopes she can have some new clothes because she and Lisa are working hard on their plan to emulate Sandie Shaw. One thing is for certain, she's determined to insist on pointy shoes for school and she is NEVER, NEVER going to have her hair cut short again!

The family have done all the usual things this holiday. There are beach trips during the day and picnics on the moors; then card games and dominoes at night – when granddad sets up the old green baize card table and nana reaches into the pantry to bring out bottles of Cream Soda, Cherry Pop and packets of crisps. But one day something happens to make the young girl feel sad. Her father asks her to take a walk along the pier with him to watch the fishing and crabbing as her little sister is quite happy building sandcastles with nana. For the first time ever she simply doesn't want to go.

'What's the matter,' her father quizzes, 'you seem in a mood?'

The young girl feels in a mood – she's not sure why –

except there's a part of her that wants to be someplace – anyplace – other than here. She sulks and stares at the ground whilst scuffing her beach shoes into the grains of sand on the concrete path.

'Come on,' her father encourages, 'it will be fun.'

The young girl reluctantly tags along, all the time thinking that she'll soon be thirteen and how she's certain Sandie Shaw doesn't go fishing with her dad – mucking up her lovely bare feet with dirty sand and spoiling her sleek bob with wind and sea spray. And it isn't fun at all – seeing the poor little fish squirming on the end of a line and having their gills ripped open and their heads chopped off!

That night she has the Z-bed to herself. Her little sister refuses to settle and has fallen asleep stuck between mum and dad. The young girl has a nightmare and wakes up trembling. She can't get the image of the fish's guts, being brutally torn away, out of her head. She feels sick. She hates being sick and always tried to avoid it. The last time she'd been really sick she was only five – it was the blueberry jam that had done it. Her dad had come into her and changed her nightdress and stayed with her until she felt better.

She begins to cry – not too loud because she doesn't want to wake everyone. The room is so silent – surely her father can hear her? The more she panics the more the tears fall and the bolder the picture in her head of the fish's blood and guts becomes. Why isn't her father coming to her? Eventually she cries herself to sleep – but when she wakes the next morning she knows something has changed. Some irrevocable shift in her relationship to her father has taken place and she has brought this about by her own free will.

Everything looks normal when she walks into the sitting room. Nana is making cups of tea; granddad is trying to get a fire going in the hearth and her father is cooking bacon in the kitchen. He smiles at her and asks if she'd like a bacon sandwich.

The young girl smiles back but it's as though she now had some worrying secret that she has to carry alone. She thinks to herself she should have seen it coming. When was the last time she sat on her father's knee and played 'round and round the garden like a teddy bear'? It was years ago! Surely all that childish stuff had belonged to her little sister for ages now. But she had wanted her dad last night for comfort – just as he had wanted her companionship earlier in the day. It was all a bit of a puzzle and for the first time ever on holiday she thinks it would be nice to be back at home in the Midlands with her school friends.

★ ★ ★

'It's difficult for humans,' Leopard sighs,

'Meaning …?'

'Well – the way you need to interpret everything. If you're simply a leopard cub a biff on the nose from your mum is just that – a biff on the nose. As for dads – they don't even figure – lazy lot of good for nothings. So that's one half of the equation knocked clean out of the picture.'

TWENTY SIX

This Is Not My Time

SIX FEET UNDER

People I should have met;
A clown
A poet
A philosopher
A beautiful bareback rider
A dancer

Believe me – there is a space in your life
where I might have been.

It didn't happen because I was holed up for years,
but you will be pleased to hear that last summer
we broke through the bedroom wall.
The cat smiled – caught in a shaft of light – and the builder,
all twenty stone of him, cried.

*I had planned other escape routes, for one, the finesse of the pen
to squeeze through a gap in the sky, but walking through the hole
in the wall was easier.*

*Oh – I have forgotten to add to my list an undertaker,
who is preferably willing to work in reverse.
I need him to dig me up – because this is not my time.*

I cannot pretend there are never days when I wish for a
physical release – when my body and mind wage war and all
I desire is an escape into infinite *peace*. Self-obliteration seems
to be the only solution. This feeling never lasts for long but I
understand why a fellow traveller might resort to such an
action. Who can say when a human being's time has come –
who has the right to presume such knowledge?

Between 2005 and 2007, three life-changing events lifted
me far away from those dark thoughts. Firstly: Matthew
taking retirement from London, secondly: the death of my
father, and thirdly: the birth of my granddaughter.

'I have to admit that was a strange period – when *time*
slipped back into this room,' Leopard concedes.

'I believe so Leopard – time's presence was palpable.'

'Are you going to tell those three stories – for the three
events?'

'I can if you like – where shall I begin?'

'With 'The Penguin Slippers' – that's my favourite
because things got a whole lot better round here after then.'

THE PENGUIN SLIPPERS
2005

The postman looked a bit bemused as he walked away from our front door. Hanging from the doorknocker was a pair of fluffy penguin slippers – size 6 – tied on with a big yellow bow. No one could possibly guess their significance.

The slippers had been a novelty purchase a few years ago. Matthew had been working away from home for many years and our thoughts were increasingly drawn to the possibility of his taking early retirement from London and building a small practice in our home town. The financial implications of this were worrying because there was no certainty of any demand locally for another psychotherapist. The counselling profession had grown exponentially since we trained, back in the 1980's, and the job market was now flooded.

'I'm going to sit by the fire and wear my penguin slippers when I manage this,' Matthew joked.

The slippers were put away and forgotten about – except during cupboard clean outs. 'Oh well – maybe one day,' we sighed.

A turning point was forced by the sudden worsening of my condition in 2004, when I became bed-bound for several months and it became apparent I would need to use a wheelchair full time. My coping reserves plummeted as I experienced the two situations I'd been most afraid of – namely not being able to see to my basic needs and a fear of abandonment. In simple terms, it was one more item to be added to *the knowing* – that list I'd been extending and editing since my realisation as a small child that life is sometimes scary.

The next ten months were tense and grim. I accepted that ethically Matthew could not suddenly abandon his London practice – he had a responsibility to his long-term clients to wind things down gently. During those months I had to face my inner demons. I didn't cope well and was often in tears and a state of panic. Those ten months felt like ten years – time certainly has some tricks to play.

So – the penguin slippers' day was a memorable event for Matthew and I. We couldn't believe that after sixteen years we were actually going to get to live together *every day*!

The saying 'absence makes the heart grow fonder' may contain a truth – but not for us. To share part of each day with my best friend is an aspect of my life I will never take for granted – bar the odd grumpy occasion when an ill wind blows through the house and we are left dazed and wondering how we managed to get so out of step.

Regarding being out of step, something strange happened on Boxing Day, 2005. I had not seen my parents for a while but they were invited for tea and I could feel my stomach tightening into a familiar knot. Would the visit pass off peaceably or would we end up umpiring a kerfuffle? I was shocked when I saw my mother – she had lost weight and seemed frail. She and my father sat companionably – like bookends – with a table of food between them, verbally appreciating the warmth of the fire, the comfort of the chairs and how nice it was to see everybody.

Later – when I was resting – my mother came and sat quietly by the bed. After a little while and having enjoyed a brief conversation she said, 'Well – do I have to go now?'

It was like an obedient child asking for an instruction on how to behave and I had never heard her speak that way before.

I stared hard at my mother's face. She had always had a smooth complexion but now it was lined. Within those lines I saw the face of my grandmother and all the past generations of women within our family. I also saw my own future and that of my daughter, my sisters and future generations stretching into infinity.

For the first time in my life I felt unafraid of death. But, perhaps of even greater importance, I sensed an emptying out of any anger I'd ever felt towards my mother. The fact that she would die – perhaps one day soon – struck me forcibly. The poet Rumi writes of a place beyond ideas of right-doing and wrong-doing. He calls the place 'the field' and it is situated outside of language, beyond our critical judgements and ruminations over the past. It is a place of unconditional love.

I gazed deep into the lines on my mother's face and saw written there the story of a little girl who had not always had an easy time.

As an only child, until the birth of her brother when she was fourteen, I do not doubt my mother was the centre of attention and surrounded by love. I had experienced the warmth and generosity of my grandparents and listened to stories about the happy times my mother spent with her own adored grandparents and extended family.

But here was a little girl who was frequently taken from her bed to stay with her grandparents because her father had come home the worse for wear due to drink. This was no doubt commonplace in many families at the time. For my grandfather there was also the trauma of having been in a terrible war and losing a brother on the battle field, and then having to spend two years in hospital after it was all over, recovering from his injuries. When I add to this the fact of his mother dying, when he was a young boy, it feels wrong to judge him harshly. However, the excessive drinking cast a shadow over my mother's childhood and it was with good reason that she sought a husband who was not a drinking man.

My grandfather, much loved by my parents, had mellowed by the time my sisters and I were born, and though this same man had always been a good grandfather to me I couldn't deny the negative consequences of his behaviour for my mother as a child, and the impact of her highly sensitive personality on our own family life.

More recently, my mother told me she developed a close relationship to her father in his final years, saying it was lovely to be able to sit and talk with him. She was sad and troubled for a long period of time after his death and maybe this was the start of things spiralling out of control at home as she lost interest in the house and began hoarding every item that passed through the front door.

The bonds of attachment and the significance of loss have a powerful effect on the mind.

'I think the Boxing Day memory is one of my favourite stories,' Leopard says.

'Why's that?'

'Well – because you're beginning to develop the capacity to combine stealth with compassion.'

I hold hands with my son's partner as we wait for the funeral cortège. We sit near the back of the church in case I need to make a quiet retreat. Wherever I go these days – even the event of my father's funeral – I feel confined in my wheelchair and need to know there is an exit door close by.

The exit door is the same door my father pushed against when I was a four-year-old. The church appears as I'd remembered – sunlight streams through the stained glass windows and the statue of Mary still wears the same beatific smile. In his later years dad had spent many hours sitting here in conversation with his saviour. Was Jesus listening and did he provide dad with all the answers he was seeking?

Question one: *'why is the world so cruel?*

My father refused to watch the news or read a newspaper in his final months. 'Adds to the worrying thoughts,' he told me whilst in respite care.

Question two: *'Is it possible for a couple to be as happy as they were when they first fell in love?'*

Did Jesus ever take a course in marriage guidance counselling?

Question three: *'Please make my daughter better – why does she have to go on being ill?'*

Back to question one on that issue dad.

A dog-eared copy of Thomas à Kempis' canonical work *The Imitation of Christ* sits on my book shelf, simply because it belonged to my father. It is one of those books he would occasionally leave on the doorstep for me to read; no doubt hoping it might give some form of reassurance. It was impossible to get annoyed with him over this, despite my having made it clear I found no personal comfort in organised religions.

'What most of all hinders heavenly consolation is that you are slow in turning yourself to prayer.'

Thus speaks Thomas à Kempis and these words reflect my father's anchor in life. As I sit in the House on the Hill I fix my eyes on the statue of Mary and hope, through all the years of visiting this place of prayer, dad found some consolation in his troubles.

The sight of my sisters as they accompany our father's coffin down the central aisle ruptures any sense of composure. My older sister holds herself together well – but with a look of such pain on her face that I begin to cry – and then I see my younger sister – head bent, tears freely falling as she walks by the coffin and I'm afraid that I'll lose it all together.

My little sister – beloved by my father – had held him all through the night as he lay dying in a hospital bed. It is impossible to express in words what this means to me. I know that she talked to him, calmed him, and soothed him. After the hell of three months of suffering in that bed, delirious – and slowly dying from a wound infection after a hip repair operation following a fall – my father's departure from this world was calm and safe. His last words to my younger sister and I had been 'I love you' – an assurance rung out from a fog of delirium as we were leaving his bedside one visit. Thanks to my sister I can be at peace knowing that the last words he heard, the last embrace he felt – echoed back, 'we love you too, always, forever, for all time.'

A New Life

One week before Dad's death.

She is tiny weighing less than five pounds. Swaddled in a blanket, and wearing a knitted pink hat, all that can be seen are two closed eyes, a button nose and rosebud mouth. She is beautiful – of course she is beautiful – she is my granddaughter.

My daughter and I swop places. It's a relief to lie on the bed after the journey. I haven't slept because tensions have been running high concerning my father's care and there have been harsh words within our family. It is such a joy to enter another hospital in another town, and a ward that beckons new life instead of encroaching death.

I hold the warm bundle and release two tiny arms from the blanket. The baby's arms make balletic movements –

stretching and waving through space. We wait for her to open her eyes – for that magical first gaze. This little one has the look of an old soul – she feels very special.

It breaks my heart that my father will not meet this newborn who is his eighth great-grandchild.

Sometimes the turn of the kaleidoscope is seismic. Any weariness I've been feeling is transformed into a revived determination to make the best of each day no matter what the difficulties. This one precious life and this one precious moment is all we ever have.

★ ★ ★

I didn't imagine I could sustain such determination by willpower or intent alone. The months leading up to my father's death had underlined for me that I had not truly erased a spiritual need from within my heart. A Catholic friend sent me some rosary beads – so akin to the ones I'd lost as a child that I was moved to tears and I found myself repeating all the Catholic prayers for the sick and dying she'd sent on request. Out of respect for my father it seemed fitting to both pray and grieve in this way, but as an answer to any personal spiritual quest Western religion had too many negative connotations for me.

'I don't know where to find an answer,' I say to Leopard.

'Perhaps you should just stop asking the question,' he replies.

It was true – despite years of trawling through so many ideas I still hadn't found any comforting notion that arrested the stone-cold fear of death which suddenly hit me as I

175

attempted to drop off to sleep each night. The major questions remained unanswered and I was still the four-year-old nervously searching under the bed and in the wardrobe for the boogie man in the night-time shadowy light.

TWENTY SEVEN

Leopard's Question
January 2009

I Google *'what is the life span of a leopard?'*

The Internet is a wondrous invention. I travel along its astral thread – once again connected to the world.

'I could have licked my PhD into shape if I'd had this!' I enthuse to Leopard. 'See – I have even carved out an identity for myself at *www.paulaburns.co.uk.* How easy it is to exist in the virtual world.'

Leopard gives one of his derisory snorts. I notice he humours me less these days.

'What's the answer?' he enquires.

'Mm …?'

'The answer to the Google thingy.'

'There are 94,600 replies,' I announce.

'I don't think I need that many predictions of my demise,' Leopard dryly retorts, as he stretches out and struggles to find a comfy position.

The creature holds his head erect and fixes me with a steely stare before asking, 'How long have we been caged up here?'

'Er – 19 years.'

'… and what is the life-span of a leopard in captivity according to your technological cosmic crystal ball?'

'21 – 23 years.'

'Then there's not much time left to finish this – you'd better get your skates on.'

2009 is proving to be one of those 'bright yellow bubble' years. In March we experience the excitement of another baby – this time a boy – and we are thrilled that my daughter now has 'one of each'. In the summer my stepdaughter has twins – a boy and a girl – a brother and sister for a little boy born just one year earlier. Matthew and I are doing very well in the grand-parenting stakes!

After many years of writing I'm also about to publish a novel entitled *Blue-Grey Island* which is in memory of my father. Started long before dad's decline it is an imagining of the inner world of a dementia sufferer. I do not know if the island of the novel is a mirror image of the place my father's mind resided during the final months of his life – but perhaps we are all destined to finally settle on our individual islands, places inhabited by the ghosts of our past and the spectral echoes of a life we once lived.

'Dad can see seagulls perched on the end of his bed,' my younger sister had told me after one hospital visit.

'Yes – that figures.'

'I don't like seagulls,' she continued, 'do you think they might be doves?'

'The doves of peace? Well – that would be comforting.'

Who knows? Dad saw many strange things – said strange things – but there was generally some basis in logical connectivity.

After one visit my son recounted a conversation that had made him smile. Dad was clearly off kilter as he rarely swore other than on the rare occasion he was very angry. A tall woman, with an abundance of wild, afro hair had walked along the central corridor by dad's ward.

'Did you see that?' dad exclaimed in a loud voice.

'What's that granddad?'

'That!' dad boomed, pointing in the woman's direction.

My son looks at the woman – hopes she can't hear through the glass partition.

'That!' dad repeats. 'What kind of a dog is that – it's like a bloody big poodle!'

Giant poodles, doves and pigeons, long-lost brothers, the urgency of factory work and needing to shave before going to church; a tableaux of characters and landmarks drawn from the past, and a plethora of new imaginings, inhabited an inner world as it came into existence moment to moment.

The theme of death – how we might imagine those last residing moments of our lives – how we might make peace with our fear – was to figure strongly in my art work and writing from here on in.

★ ★ ★

Over twenty years plus, since my becoming ill, the garden still maps our world. Down came an old hut to make way for a sunny patio, and a new little shed with a ceramic representation of Sun hung on the door.

'You're smiling a lot on that plaque,' Moon remarks, glancing down.

'Well – it's not for real – is it?' Sun snaps. 'I do my best to shine for the humans but I'd be lost without the clouds to doze behind.'

The shed is packed with toys for our grandchildren, five of whom are under the age of six. Leopard feels rejuvenated since the arrival of his new playmates. A joyful heart wins over a failing body – most of the time.

My ability to walk more than a few steps unassisted didn't return.

Leopard snarled, 'this cage is totally made of bricks – there are not even bars!'

I won't bore you with tales of the hammering of walls coming down and the widening of doorways – which began with the hole in the wall back in 2007 and continued through the entire house, 'till it was disabled accessible from the ground floor all the way up to the attic. But I will mention the pleasure of seeing Sun's light entering previously gloomy rooms – how it bounced off ceilings and newly laid laminate flooring and sparkled on mirrors.

My spirit child doesn't normally enter the house, but on this occasion she popped her head round the patio door.

'How does the space grow?' she repeats her question.

'It just does,' I reply, 'like the space inside your heart. Infinity can only be grasped through love.'

She raises an eyebrow. 'Still attached to words I see?'

'I'm afraid so – can't quite seem to kick the habit.'

The allure of words is hard to resist but I no longer consult the daily oracle. Even Sun has decided to lay off for a while after a huge commotion with Moon.

Thinking back, the conflict began in June – 2006. Sun had become quite literate over the years – almost level-pegging with her sister. The reading of headlines no longer posed a problem.

INTERPLANETARY ESTATE AGENTS CALL ON INVESTORS TO ASK FOR THE MOON.
The Guardian – June 15th – 2006

'See what they're up to now,' Sun announced to unsuspecting Moon, 'the humans are selling bits of you.'

Moon felt edgy. Her little naps, snatched from the moments when clouds obscure the humans' view of her, were haunted by dreams within which she shed gallons of tears. She couldn't discern why she was crying but in her dream the tears became frozen lakes – preserved beneath her lunar dust. On discovering this bounty the humans reignited their desire to inhabit her body.

'They know, they know!' she screamed at Sun.

'Know what?'

'They know about the water! They're going to use me as some extra-terrestrial filling station so they can explore further into deeper space.'

Sun conceded that carrying water to Moon was expensive – just a few extra pints (contributing to the weight) could add one hundred thousand pounds to a rocket's fuel bill. Even so, she resisted the spiteful urge to feed her sister's paranoia.

'Don't be daft,' she scolded, 'you said yourself no one's really interested in you anymore. You should be careful what you ask for.'

Things quietened down for a while, but in 2007 it all kicked off again. Moon honed in on a headline that plunged her into a torrent of anger towards Sun. In Moon's view her sister was now responsible for every distressing situation.

PLUNDERING THE MOON

'THE NEW SPACE RACE ISN'T FOCUSED ON SCIENCE OR DISCOVERY, BUT IS ABOUT EXPLOITING LUNAR MINERALS.'
The Guardian – October 27th – 2007

Leopard and I crawled under the duvet. We could still hear Moon screeching at Sun – some days it felt like the whole world was screeching.

'See what you've done now,' Moon wailed. 'I tried to tell you before – all that stupid dancing causes havoc. Oh – I want to be anonymous again. I know you tried to warn me – celebrity is horrible. I want to be forgotten!'

'Bet she doesn't mean it,' I whispered to Leopard. 'No one really wants to be forgotten.'

'What happened to the 'dry bones and ashes' whine?' Sun snapped, 'I thought you wanted to be special?'

The year 2020 currently looms in Moon's mind. This is the year China aims to put a citizen on Moon and the US also plan a return. But Moon feels this visit is suspect – driven by something sinister.

'If you'd just stop jigging about there wouldn't be any lunar dust,' she pleads with her sister.

At times, Sun is pure arrogance. In recent years she has become further inflated by her self-education. Sun has learnt the power of words to do harm as well as good.

'Well,' she countered, 'they don't call it moon dust – it's called He-3 and if the humans can perfect fusion technology your moon dust could provide them with clean energy. And …' she continues, raising her voice above Moon's wailing, 'seeing as the dust is deposited because of my dancing – well – you'd be of no interest at all if it wasn't for me!'

'You're mean – I hate you!' Moon screams even louder. 'You know full well it will involve ripping up my body surface to the depth of a metre … oh no – what is a metre?'

'Not deep enough to get to your heart, sister dear,' Sun pacifies, 'definitely not deep enough get to your soul.'

TWENTY EIGHT

2012
The Daughters of Diogenes

Soon after our father's death my younger sister and her family emigrated to New Zealand. We wondered how our mother would cope with their leaving because her relationship with my sister and her young children was fairly close. But mum surprised us by adjusting really well.

Now that mum had full dominion over her home all that seemed required was the personal space to live her life exactly as she wanted. In truth, this was all she had desired for years – as we were informed in no uncertain terms whenever the opportunity arose. This request, that had been so painful and problematic when our father was alive, now seemed perfectly reasonable and my older sister and I agree to take it in turns to deliver the shopping and make regular phone calls. My sister also decides to help out with the household chores – on this score she draws the short straw.

Because of my physical limitations it falls to Matthew to

deal with the shopping but he doesn't seem to mind. As her only remaining blood relative he'd had full responsibility for his mother who lived to be one hundred and three. Every night, for over twenty years, Matthew rang Vera for a chat – he never missed a phone call despite working evenings. After she dies we can't get used to not making that phone call.

In some respects my mother is low maintenance but on another level the stress is building. Vera had been meticulous; her home, her person, her grasp of household accounts all had a sense of order. In comparison, my mother's understandable need for non-interference creates a level of chaos – or that's how it seems to our perceptions which are fuelled by a desire for a general level of organisation. The hoarding began long before my father's decline into vascular dementia. Everything that entered the house was tenaciously held onto because it might be 'useful' and over the years our mother's perceptions have become intransigently rooted within a war-time mentality.

Collections begin to grow, such as: the backs of cereal packets and cardboard wrappers on ready meals (we are assured these make good bookmarks): clothes: books: bric-a-brac: newspapers: cuddly toys and postcards. Everything comes in multiples. It reaches a point where I can no longer negotiate a path down the hallway in my wheelchair. There has not been a free chair to sit on for years, but it's particularly upsetting to see our father's old armchair in the corner of the dining room, replete with its saggy springs, now piled high with books and clothes.

The dining room, which looks out onto the garden, is the only day room our parents occupied in their later years, as the front lounge became an overspill terminal for surplus books and clothes. There isn't an inch of space on the dining room table as we attempt to sort an increasingly complex regime of medication. In many respects we accept that our mother has a right to live as she wants – the problem lies within ourselves because we desire some change or at least to be met half-way. We see danger where she perceives none – where we see grime and disorder our mother envisions a familiar nest.

From 2007 until 2012 we aim to keep mum afloat at home. *Five years* – another five puffs of dandelion floss. Such a period of time can seem fleeting when viewed in retrospect but during those years tasks of a repetitive nature came to dominate the pattern of our lives. If I were to paint that pattern it would be an infinite number of circles in monochrome – intersected by a few flashes of red.

So, every week the trip to Marks and Spencer's to buy the little meals in the special cardboard wrappers mum likes, and a Swiss roll in its box with a sticker announcing *special offer – two for the price of one* – which always sparks a debate. But each week the meals from the previous week's shopping are removed from the fridge and replaced with fresh ones. It becomes impossible to encourage mum to eat at all. It's not that she lacks appetite but as her short term memory loss escalates she's unable to process essential tasks, like preparing and cooking food, and doesn't remember if she's eaten.

The cooker becomes a hazard as it is used as yet another surface to put items on, and tea towels and newspapers are left perilously close to the gas ring. A microwave and toaster isn't a possible alternative because mum's afraid of 'new machinery'. She's overwhelmed by an anxiety focused on things 'going up in a blue light'. We try ready-made sandwiches and other ploys to encourage her to eat but nothing works. All of this time our mother is resolutely independent and refuses to consider outside help. We have to admire her spirit – gaining an insight into a feisty personality that made her fearless whilst attending to her nursing duties during the blitz in the Second World War – but just now she's more in danger of burning the house down than falling bombs.

We are at our wits end but social services are adamant – there's nothing to be done because our mother has performed OK on 'the test' – so why should we be worried? She can – after all – remember the name of the Prime Minister.

Years roll by. Mum wears the same clothes week on week and every single thing in the house has become an object of intense attachment. Nothing can be moved and nothing can be cleaned without causing immense agitation. Dickens' tale of Miss Havisham pales into insignificance in comparison and we are truly afraid of the fire hazard. Mum has taken to smoking and an ominous burnt patch appears on her beloved joggers which she obstinately refuses to relinquish to the heinous threat of my sister's washing machine.

The social worker persists that mum can still make her own decisions – taken in by her client's account of a day structured by routine and confidently delivered by rote. Well – it's sweet that mum totters out into the garden to feed the mice and the birds – the problem is she's not feeding herself – and furthermore, a *client* is an individual a social worker occasionally visits but a *mother* is an individual lodged in our hearts despite the difficulties. The act of 'doing one's duty' is more complex than we're generally prepared for.

The emergency call pendant hangs forgotten by the bed

and every time I visit I ask mum where this essential device is and why she doesn't wear it. She always tells me she's removed it because she's about to wash her hair. I go through the drill dozens of times but she can't remember the instructions.

'But what if I'm in the garden feeding the birds?' she says.

'It's important to wear the pendant all the time Mum – what if you fall over out there?'

'Oh yes – I know – but I was just about to wash my hair.'

Other than one of us being with our mother every day it's like abandoning her to her fate.

One lunch-time the social worker finds her client still in bed – a wet bed – not having had a warm drink or taken her medication. Some recognition of the real extent of the problem begins to dawn.

We do not want our mother to have to leave her home and be taken into care but she is totally resistant to a reasonable conversation about carers and additional help, and her memory is so poor that she would not remember a conversation that agreed to a care plan anyway. As phone calls only exist within the moment, leaving no trace within her mind, she must feel abandoned despite our vigilance.

My sister and I walk a tightrope over feelings of sadness, frustration and anger. Where does the basic human right to live as one pleases begin and end? Leaving our mother to her own devices is beginning to feel like child neglect.

'The hoarding – it's called Diogenes syndrome,' I say to my sister.

'I know,' she sighs, 'it's on the internet. It seems strange that the psychiatrist hasn't mentioned the condition at all.'

The party line seems to be to wait and see – wait for the

inevitable accident. Mum will either have a fall or burn the house down. This is the best the authorities can come up with. The precarious 'solution' isn't acceptable to our family – we've already been through the anguish of witnessing one parent die from the complications of a hip fracture following a fall.

A weird thought begins to dawn. Perhaps we are going to have kidnap our mother from the clutches of social services, as we're convinced that the powers set up by the State to protect the elderly are inadvertently pushing her into a decline. It isn't that the social worker is uncaring or not bothered but she has to deliver a particular script and is in a difficult position. There are no doubt relatives who want to free themselves of a burden and this has to be taken into account. But we are indignant, 'isn't it obvious we don't fall into that category?' we protest. 'Finding care will after all mean selling the house. If we were duplicitous wouldn't we just let the situation play out and collect our inheritance at the end point?'

'This is wearing,' I say to Leopard.

'Yes – you don't learn ethics from a text book.'

I begin to research care homes and find one close to where my sister and I live. I like the feel of the place because there is nothing institutionalized about the atmosphere. Our mother can have a large, sunny room at the front of the house. A little dog nudges up close as the manager tells me that residents can have breakfast in their rooms – there are no strict rules and regulations.

'My mother would love this little dog,' I remark, thinking

of how lonely she has been since her own dog died a couple of years ago.

'Then she can have her,' the manager smiles – I'll take the dog with me when I visit.'

I can't believe our luck; a homely care home with a resident pet – right on our doorstep.

'Can I take your photo?' I ask the dog.

'Woof!'

'Well that's good, because I've got a hell of a lot of persuading to do to pull this off.'

We're amazed that mum agrees to take 'a little holiday'. In our hearts we know it's not going to be respite care – that if she settles it will need to be a permanent arrangement. The trouble is she immediately forgets about the visit from the nice lady with the 'lovely little dog'. I've pinned the dog's photo to mum's notice board but it fails to jog her virtually non-existent short term memory.

My sister and I are in a quandary.

'I can't do it,' my sister declares, 'what if she changes her mind, what if she gets agitated. She'll never forgive us.'

'I can't face it either.'

It feels like back to the drawing board but the care home manager comes to the rescue.

When we arrive at the home to find mum settled in her room, washed and changed and not seeming overtly put out, it's as though a miracle has taken place.

'How did you do it?' we ask.

'I just kind of scooped her up.'

'What – she came willingly?'

'Well, I didn't give her too much time to discuss it, but really – she's fine.'

Mum *did* seem fine. She fussed the little dog which already had a basket in her room and told one of the carers what she'd like for her tea from the multiple choice menu. It was all so comfortable and amiable that I was beginning to feel I wouldn't mind moving in for a rest myself!

'Well it's very nice here,' Mum smiles, 'but I'm only here for a fortnight you understand – it's just for a little holiday.'

Those words were to come back to haunt us because it's what Mum says every time we visit. She's fairly happy and contented, extremely well physically and has put on weight. She likes her room and adores Snowy the cat who has taken up residence on her bed (after the little dog mysteriously disappeared one day). But over a year later – within a memory that is shot to bits – our mother's fully aware she's been spirited away from her home and for reasons she can't comprehend has never returned. She doesn't remember her actual house and talks about once living in a bungalow. She knows she has left something behind – a life she had before the present moment – but it's all hazy. Her long term memory is fully intact and she can recall and talk about the early and middle years of her life, but something in those recollections is askew.

Mum recounts that we were a very happy family, dad and she and us three girls. By all accounts there was *no* tension, *no* unhappiness – we all did 'really well together'. I think to myself, 'I would like some of that memory – would have loved to *really* live it'.

Perhaps when I'm old I'll be blessed to live in a re-figured inner world and all the issues I feel guilty about, and things I wish I'd done better, will simply melt away. What bliss!

CHAPTER TWENTY NINE

2012
Sky Path

The year isn't totally consumed by elder care. Art comes to the rescue and provides an alternative focus when I become involved in a joint installation project with an artist friend.

We are fortunate in having an inspirational location for the installation within the grounds of a national organic garden. Our plan is to install a walkway with five gates – composed of screens made from loosely hung ribbons. The ribbons will be based upon the colours and symbolism of Tibetan prayer flags.

Matthew and I visit the garden in winter. The layout lends itself to an oriental theme and my co-artist and I eventually settle on a pergola from which to hang the installation. The next eight months are to be spent sourcing ribbons in the correct shade of Tibetan colours (yellow, green, red, white and blue) and exploring themes within the symbolism. We imagine the ribbons as five gate ways within a pathway which will take visitors on an inner journey, beginning with yellow (the solidity of earth) through water, fire and air to blue (the huge expanse of sky and heaven, known as 'the void') .

The project chimes with another interest that is gaining momentum. We live in a free associative age; a poem (Mary Oliver's *Wild Geese*) is referenced on a web blog alongside the mention of a Vietnamese Zen Buddhist monk named Thich Nhat Hanh. I read Mary Oliver's collection of poetry and one of Thich Nhat Hanh's books entitled *Peace is Every Step* and experience an intuition that I've stumbled on a path that might lead *home*.

Leopard sighs, 'I hope this isn't going to be another quest?'

'I'm partial to those aren't I?' I laugh, 'but it feels good to have a *sense of knowing* that isn't laced with fear.'

'Does it involve philosophy?' Leopard persists.

'Er … a bit – I guess – well yes, but only if you're that way inclined – it mainly involves just sitting quietly – not grasping and attaching to thoughts – and letting things *just be*.'

Leopard knows me too well and he's right to be wary. I can't pretend the ongoing experience is trouble free – though the trouble is self-induced. The associated reading material has evolved into a library exceeding a hundred books – requiring the acquisition of more shelves.

'You do realise all this investigation might add to the yapping?' Leopard cautions.

'I know – but there's something about the practice that draws me in. There is nothing final or even essential in all the written words – the words just point to the practice – nothing more.'

Leopard fixes me with a look that signals disbelief. 'So why do you go on buying the books?'

'Well – as you're aware – it's an addiction I'm working on.'

'I won't believe you,' Leopard challenges, 'until you burn the lot.'

'Phew! – I've a long way to go – I've still got a big attachment to words.'

'And what would your Zen masters say to that?'

'Probably that by standing in a pile of ashes, that was once all the words we've ever taken in, we finally realise that everything we need to be happy is right here, right now. We don't need to be constantly searching and we definitely don't need to be reading thousands of words.'

'You're not going to start giving out Zen speak are you? You do realise how irritating it is when a lay person sounds like a ventriloquist Zen master's dummy?'

'I promise – double promise – I just need to keep this simple.'

Sky Path is installed in July, and in August Matthew and I spend a sunny day filming the ribbon gateways and celebrating my sixtieth birthday. We are discreet observers – interested in the varied response of visitors to the garden.

It seems that the different responses echo the many ways human beings walk through their lives.

Some visitors are pissed off with the ribbons! They have to pass through the pathway to reach another part of the garden and swipe their way through the dangling obstruction with great irritation.

'Why on earth have they put this here?' one women complains.

Others walk through slowly, gently parting the ribbons and feeling their silky texture. No hurry.

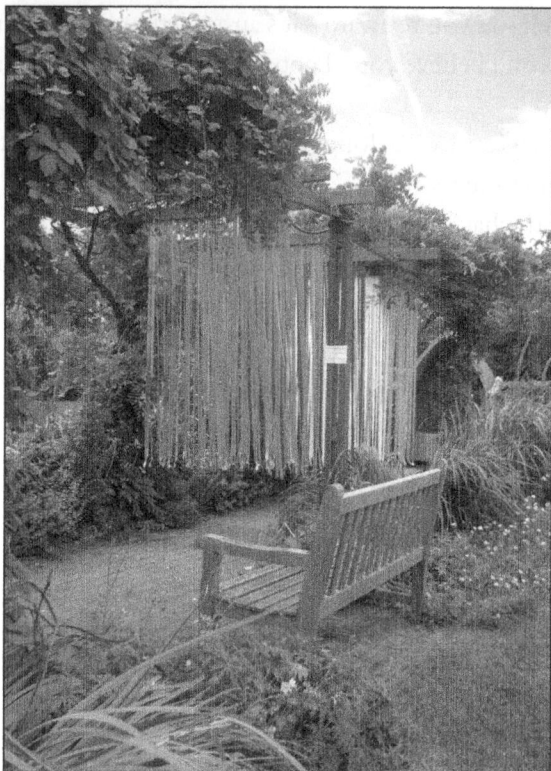

Sky Path

But the one scene we request to recreate in film is the response of a group of young children. They joyfully run back and forth through the ribbons with no particular sense of linear progression – which is how I perceive the pathway.

'What did it make you think of?' I ask one little girl, who is breathless with excitement.

'Oh – it's like running through a rainbow,' she smiles.

THIRTY

Another self-portrait

'Gravity has taken its toll,' I say to Leopard.

He yawns and paws at the dressing up box. 'Just don't look in the mirror,' he suggests.

'Well – the camera is a mirror and there's no doubt I look like an elderly plumped up Peppa Pig in this pink ballet tutu!'

'Best try the black then – it'll be slimming.'

I wonder within myself what it is I'm trying to convey? Ten years ago I could still walk from the camera (set up on its tripod) to the far side of the room. Not any more – not without a Zimmer frame. If I lean against the door I can manage a standing position for thirty seconds; there is just enough time to traverse the floor and pose before the auto-timer clicks and the lens shoot. I feel like a puppet strung up against the door frame – arms and legs flung out akimbo. I attempt to adopt the classical fifth ballet position. All of the ballet positions are indelibly etched into my brain. For a few seconds, trembling limbs seem able to sustain a miraculous sense of balance and poise.

There is a click and a flash before I grasp onto the walking frame to steady myself. I call Matthew and we pose for a celebratory sixtieth birthday photo. All of the images are very different to the ones I took a decade ago. When I look for some kind of personal statement in them the only picture I can title is the one of Matthew and I together. I write the words *'the person who really holds me up'* on the back of the photo.

THIRTY ONE

2013
This used to be my Home

The estate where I grew up is not so far away from my present home and sometimes nostalgia dictates that Matthew and I take a drive past the house and garden where I took my first steps; rode my first bike and made petal perfume with Lisa. A short detour takes me to the second house we lived in, opposite the humpty dumpty fields, and then a drive round the corner and up a hill brings me to the third and final home within which my parents were to see out their days.

This third dwelling, where I lived between the ages of thirteen to eighteen, must now be sold in order to fund our mother's care home fees. My sister and I are overwhelmed by the task in hand and my younger sister fretful that she is not around to help us.

In the beginning our parents had very few possessions. If I close my eyes it's easy to visualize our first home and to step through the portal of time connecting the past to the present.

'Wait!' Leopard interrupts, making me jump. 'There's nothing wrong with nostalgia but it does have a tendency to make humans repeat themselves.'

'I just need to return to the child's story for a couple of pages Leopard. This is how humans uncover memory. A story doesn't necessarily unfurl in one linear time frame after another. Clearing my mother's house has made me question when the storm clouds really began.'

* * *

The seven year old skips from room to room. The kitchen is clean and tidy and the dining and sitting rooms contain just the required amount of furniture – there is no clutter.

Lisa knocks at the child's kitchen door, which opens out onto the wash house and garage. All of this is perceived as play space by the children. The garage is stuffed with toys and bikes. There is a large doll's pram and – best of all – a Bronco sit-on metal pedal horse. The horse is painted white and grey and has a red and gold saddle. None of the other children in the road have such a horse. In the corner of the wash house there's some new machine with a mangle that magically squeezes the water out of the laundry, but it's of less importance than her father's gardening tools and a rack of wellies and outdoor shoes.

Some of her friends' mothers use their wash houses to cook in, making them a no-go-area. The little girl thinks that's a waste of good play space, especially when it rains and it's too wet to play in the street.

'What shall we play,' Lisa demands, barging into the kitchen.

The child ponders for a moment. Her mother has popped to the shops and they have the place to themselves. Her father's around somewhere – but he's bound to be in the garden.

'Special recipes?' she suggests.

Lisa grins. Nothing is ever ordinary with her playmate, it's always *special* this or *magic* that but seeing as food's involved she decides to let it go without teasing.

'Ok – what shall we make?'

The child drags a kitchen stool over to a high cupboard and after a bit of a debate the two friends start off with Weetabix with honey liberally poured over the top.

'It's too dry,' Lisa moans, 'what else have you got?'

The child climbs back onto the stool and peers into the kitchen cupboard. 'Do you think condensed milk would be good?'

Lisa pulls a face, 'well – only if you've got hundreds and thousands.'

'Of course we have,' the child replies with an air of superiority, 'and chocolate strands and silver balls … and oh – look – there's this green stuff and cherry things.'

'Let's try the lot!' Lisa enthuses.

Later, the child feels tearful remembering her father had come in just at the point Lisa was grappling with a can opener. He gave them a right telling off but the child knew it was because he'd once cut his hand on the opener and had to have stitches. It was fear that had made him shout at her. Lisa was sent home and she'd been left to clear up on her own.

'I want that worktop cleaned just like it was before you messed up, or your mum will be cross,' her dad had grumbled, but later he'd given her a little hug and she'd sat in the garden with milk and biscuits and watched him weeding.

The little girl is not short of toys. The resident dolls and teddies are neatly lined up on her bed and her favourite story books, Milly-Molly-Mandy: Teddy-Tar: Noddy: Hans Christian Anderson and Peter Pan are stacked on the book shelf. Just at the moment she's not keen on Noddy because she doesn't like the pictures of trees with faces. Last week, when she'd walked back from Brownies with her friends, the trees had looked scary because it was getting dark. She hadn't told any of the other children because she didn't want to be teased but she'd been really frightened!

The latest acquisition is a blue teddy bear. The teddy bear is special because he is a prize for winning a race at school. It wasn't that the headmaster had shaken her hand and said, 'here's a blue teddy bear for winning the race.' No – he'd presented her with a piece of paper that was a token allowing her to choose whatever she liked from the toy shop up town. Her father was very proud that she'd won the race and said she could choose whatever she liked.

The toy shop is usually far too expensive to buy anything from – though the child and her mother like to window shop, especially as it is next door to a pet shop. Sometimes there are kittens and puppies in the pet shop window, all whimpering and jumping up at the glass pane, wanting to be taken home. Inside, the shop is full of cages, housing rabbits and guinea pigs, hamsters and mice. A blue and yellow parrot perches on a stand and shrieks, 'who's a pretty Polly,' whenever it hears the tinkle of the bell as the shop door swings open.

The child thinks she is very lucky because they have loads of pets at home. It's true the pretty, green budgerigar just twitters in its cage despite her granddad's assurance it could be taught to talk just like a parrot, and her mother inexplicably goes into hysterics every time her father frees the bird from its cage to have a fly around the sitting room because she has a phobia about feathers, but most of the time their family pets are a source of pleasure and affection.

One of the reasons the wash house is tidy just now is because it's warm enough for the rabbits and guinea pigs to be outside. In the winter they will be brought inside and this is another reason the child is glad her mother only cooks in the kitchen. The little creatures' noses are always twitching and the child thinks they wouldn't like the smell of boiling cabbage and meat and dumpling stew … especially rabbit stew … that would be terrible for a pet rabbit to smell!

That summer they'd had a new litter of baby rabbits and her father promised she could hold one as soon as the babies opened their eyes. Her dad knew all about animals and when they went on walks he explained about not touching or disturbing the eggs in a bird's nest because the mother bird would go away and not come back.

When they went to exchange the prize token the little girl and her mother had looked longingly at a litter of puppies in the pet shop window. Just recently, one of their two dogs had died and her father was still sad, but he'd asked her mother to be sure not to bring any more animals home.

'Do you promise you won't let mum bring another pet home?' he'd whispered to the child, with a bit of a smile – as though he half-expected her mum to not keep her word.

The child had a little think. She and Lisa were always making promises when they wanted to keep a secret and shared an assortment of words they recited in a solemn tone of voice – such as 'Brownies' honour' – but that didn't sound quite grown-up enough for this kind of promise.

'Cross my heart and hope to die,' she beamed.

'Well – I guess we'll just buy a couple of bags of rabbit food,' her mother had compromised before they went next door to look at the toys. After much deliberation a decision had to be made between a wooden bracelet painted in bright colours or the blue bear. The child had pointed to the little blue teddy – sat on a shelf all by himself.

'He wants to come home with me,' she'd insisted.

'All right – one more for the collection,' her mother agreed, 'now let's be quick or we'll miss the bus and be late for tea.'

The following spring, six months after the child's eighth birthday, a coach built pram occupies an entire corner of the sitting room. She is excited – gives it a little push and places a cuddly toy next to the pile of nappies and baby clothes that are neatly folded on the mattress. The small bedroom, recently decorated with pretty wallpaper (colourful baskets of flowers on a black background) is to be vacated to make way for the new baby's cot.

Her father had looked quite nervous when telling her the news. He'd sat on the edge of her bed and began with, 'I have a very exciting thing to tell you.'

The child had looked at him wide-eyed. 'Is it a secret – I know how to keep a secret.'

'Well it can be a secret for now if you like.'

'I think the secret might be a new puppy?' she'd then suggested – as this was the most exciting possibility she could think of.

'Much better than a puppy,' her father had laughed, 'you're going to have a new baby brother or sister.'

The child had gone quiet for a little while – taking the news in. 'Will the baby want my bedroom?' she'd asked, not wanting to relinquish the new wallpaper. When she stared at the pattern in the semi-darkness it was almost like seeing the floating bubbles of light that were proving much harder to conjure up than when she was small.

'You'll still be able to play in here,' her father had reassured, 'the baby won't take up much room.'

The child decided she didn't mind too much – it meant she would once more share a bedroom with her older sister and this was a bonus giving her a ringside seat onto the rituals of preparing to go out on a date and other mysteries of teenage life. On the whole she is happy within her world of home, garden, school and adventures beyond, when she is allowed to play in 'the bushes' with her friends or walk down the road to buy sweets at the local shop.

The house is not so tidy once her little sister comes along because as the child discovers babies need a lot of *stuff.* Also her mother struggles to stay calm – there's a whiff of heightened tension in the air.

'So that's when the storm clouds began to gather!' Leopard leaps up and punches at the air with his paw.

'No, I don't think so Leopard – I would include this period of time within the happier years.'

The nine-year-old's world is expanding and she has ballet, swimming, brownies, roller skating and Sunday school outings to occupy her. Most of her time is spent out of the house – not in it.

When she is ten she sits at the dining room table and works on her progress papers. The child knows it's really important to score a high mark on the papers if she's to pass the eleven plus. Everything about her world is changing fast and very soon her family will be moving house and she will be going to a new school. Her father promises she can have a full size bike when she's eleven – it doesn't matter whether she passes for the grammar school or not – the new bike is for definite.

'You didn't mention the bike when you told the story before?' Leopard quizzes.

'No – I'd forgotten. But I can see it clearly now. It had some fancy words stencilled on the frame in red and gold letters.'

Moving from her familiar home is strange but once the child knows she is going to the grammar school she accepts the changes. At least Lisa will be joining her but all of her other friends are going to a different school. Even so, she can't help but notice that the next house is a bit ramshackle and very small. Things feel cramped but her parents say they won't be living there for long – it's just while they save up.

Several months later the child is enjoying her new school. It's a three mile bike ride to get there and she feels very grown-up cycling the distance on her big bike. It doesn't seem long since she fell off her first tricycle and cut her knee so badly it left a big circle of blood on the pavement.

In a few weeks time the family will be moving house once again.

'It's our very own home,' her mother explained, 'we won't have to pay rent to dad's works.'

The child is excited because the garden backs onto fields with grazing cattle, and there is a farmhouse in the distance about which she is already making up stories. In actual fact the new home is a modest three bedroom semi, but since starting the local grammar school the child has become conscious of difference. Some niggling sense of inferiority is pushing her into painting her future home as being grander than it really is.

Despite the grammar school system operating as the great equaliser she's aware that many of her new friends live in private houses in upmarket locations – but she's part of a motley group, the composition of which staggers the two extremes of the wealthy and the not so well off. One friend lives in a pre-fab on a large council estate whilst another lives in a huge white house that seems luxurious in comparison.

'What about the special friend?' Leopard asks. 'What sort of house did she live in?'

'You mean the one whose mum made thrifty dinners? Her house was just like ours – only *tidy*.'

'We're moving into a really nice house,' the child tells her classmate from the white residence.

The classmate's older sister is icing a Christmas cake and the child thinks that the block of fondant icing – all white and smooth – looks like the external walls of the luxurious house.

But the cake, prestigiously placed on a silver board, is not so inviting as the cups of tea and mountains of toast on offer when she visits her friend who lives on the council estate.

To reach the estate she has to cycle down an alleyway. At first the child is afraid because the alley cuts through overgrown trees and bushes and the estate has a reputation for unruly behaviour. But it all feels different once inside her friend's house. Everyone crams into the kitchen (her friend has five siblings) where they chat, whilst perched on the kitchen worktops. The children's mum is warm and friendly, and no one seems to mind about the grandfather who isn't quite in his right mind and wanders in and out telling bad jokes and disjointed stories about a past life in Ireland.

The child remembers her father recounting the story of how his family had come to England from Ireland.

'My dad had to share a house with thirteen people – there were nine children – that's three more than six.'

'It's Ok having lots of brothers and sisters,' her friend replies, 'just gets a bit crowded sometimes.'

'Mm … dad only had one brother and sister – I wonder who all the other children were? Do you know – lots of the children he went to school with had no shoes – they had to walk in bare feet.'

'There you go,' her friend's mother joins in. 'You have to count your blessings in this life. You kids are luckier than you realise.'

The child knows this is true. Her dad had told her how his father was traumatised in the Second World War because he'd been trapped at sea, when all the cargo ships were being sunk by submarines. Every morning, before school, her dad had needed to help his father home from his new job as a night watchman – because her grandfather was ill with asthma and bad nerves and often struggled to breathe.

Cycling freely, down the country lanes to get to school, the child thought she was fortunate in comparison to her dad.

A sense of clarity begins to form within the child's thoughts. One of her classmates lives in a beautiful new house. It stands all on its own (this world of detached as opposed to semi-detached is a new phenomenon). But there is no sign of a dad – and after a while it becomes clear that something unspeakably horrible had happened in the garage of the beautiful home and that her friend's father had died as a result.

What with the shocking story and the lack of tea and toast at the luxurious white house the child begins to form the view that the outside of a home doesn't matter one jot – it's what happens on the inside that matters. And anyway, she feels phoney talking about her 'nice new house' – ashamed of the exaggerated boasting. Soon after moving in, she's acutely aware of a sense of unease. Something is happening on the inside of their home that's making her feel insecure and uncertain. It's as though a wave of unrest has taken hold and rises higher and higher. The child is afraid the wave will take her up in its path, swirl her around and pull her under.

'So is this the point,' Leopard tentatively suggests, 'is this where the difficulty began?'

'Maybe. You could say I experienced a heightened sensitivity to a pre-existing problem.'

'Is it part of the story?'

'Yes.'

'How many pages worth and should I sit or lie down?'

'I would lie down – you can have a little snooze if you like.'

★ ★ ★

The wave of unrest, which the child can only think of as *the noise,* had not been so apparent when they lived in the avenue. Living in a friendly environment had meant there were mitigating circumstances that prevented *the noise* from filling their entire space.

Lisa's mum had been too good a neighbour – a friendly, warm hearted woman – for her mother to fall out with. There's no doubt that the fact of Lisa's naughty little brother throwing stones at the child's baby sister's pram had induced annoyance but there was never a row.

Mrs Timmons, whose house directly adjoined at a pivotal point, namely *the fireplace*, was also a friend who her mother enjoyed going to the local theatre with. But the connected fireplaces had posed a problem. The child recollects that her mother had made more noise complaining about Mrs Timmons' perpetual poking of her hearth than the sound produced by the poking itself.

'Can you hear that poker!' her mother exclaimed in exasperation. 'Why does anyone need to poke a fire like that?'

The ice cream man was not so lucky.

'Your mum told the ice-cream man off,' a little friend teased. 'She says the noise of the jingles wakes your baby sister.'

The local butcher received short shrift too. The child longed to sink into the floor when her mother implied the 'best' mince didn't look like best mince at all. It was even worse when she was sent to do the errand on her own. 'Make sure you ask the butcher for *best mince*,' her mother demanded, 'else it won't be any good.'

But now – when it comes down to the irritating and annoying aspects of other people's quirks and foibles – the tables have been reversed. Their new neighbours are a quiet, middle-aged couple who have no children of their own.

Mr Farley likes to do his garden – very quietly – and his watercolour landscape painting – very quietly. Quietly … quietly … quietly … and into this peaceful atmosphere the child's family has descended, with a menagerie of animals plus all their human family squabbles. They have destroyed Mr and Mrs Farley's peace and Mrs Farley – who has a tendency to speak her mind – frequently tells them so!

The child has sympathy for her new neighbours. Some mornings, when she wakes early, she likes to creep out into the garden. There is a loose spoke in the top fence which she removes so that she can climb through into the fields. Then she takes a walk and lies down in the grass – looking up at the sky – the blue, blue sky and the birds gently swooping down. There is a magical sound of silence – which isn't a total lack of sound – but it is the sound of peace and she thinks to herself how poor Mr Farley would probably never enjoy that sound again, not while her family were living next door.

Naturally her mother has a conflicting narrative. The Farleys are unreasonable and spoilt and what's more Mrs Farley puts the vacuum cleaner on at the ungodly hour of 7.30am *every* morning! Who in their right mind cleans at that time of day and how can there be any dirt when there's no-one to make a mess!

211

The child has to admit their own house is more in need of a vacuum cleaner. The guinea pigs have taken up residence in the front sitting room, scattering sawdust and straw all over the carpet. There's also been a run on 'unsuitable puppies' recently. The latest resident puppy lives behind the fireguard in the dining room until the decision is made to return the 'irritating, whimpering bundle' to its original owner. The child is instructed to return the puppy on her own so her friend from the white house kindly offers to pop the confused animal into the large wicker basket, attached to the front of her bike, and to accompany her mortified class mate. The child had cried and begged her mother to be allowed to keep the little black spaniel, and feels awkward having to explain its 'unsuitable nature' to the original owner.

The trouble is the puppy made a *noise*!

The child's grandfather is fond of tongue twisters and now she has a new one for him. *It's possible to make more noise/ complaining about a noise/ than the noise/ the actual noise/ makes itself.*

Mrs Farley was to have the last word. Years later – when the child is grown, having turned eighteen and now living away from home, she runs into Mrs Farley in town. Mrs Farley grabs hold of her – not in an unfriendly way, but with the determination of someone who has something important to say.

'How did you stand it?' she says, her face crumpling with the intensity of the thought she must convey. 'How did you stand living in all that *noise*? It killed Mr Farley, you know?'

The eighteen-year-old wobbles – knocked sideways by the force of words.

'I'm sorry,' she says, 'I'm really very sorry,' and walks away.

She feels upset and embarrassed – yet strangely vindicated. It seemed unlikely that her mother had actually killed Mr Farley – after all nobody else had died – so that had to be an exaggeration, didn't it? But at least someone from the outside world had the measure of what she'd been up against as a child. Mr Farley must have known exactly what she was feeling as he watched her from his painting studio; a young girl from next door slipping the loose pole in the garden fence and escaping into the wide, blue sky.

★ ★ ★

When the eighteen-year-old thinks back she has to admit the thing she remembers most (from the previous six years) *is* raised voices and the various ways in which she had tried to escape the fall out. In addition to her early morning walks there had been visits to friends' houses, visits to the home of a church member who took her under his wing, weekends away babysitting for her maths teacher who lived in an idyllic setting beside a canal and visiting her sister who was now married with twins. Eventually, she had sought the ultimate escape in college and leaving home.

And yet … a home isn't simply geography. Over the coming years the critical eighteen-year-old will continue to set aside a room in her mind which contains everything about her parents she still loves and she will find herself returning to that room in times of trouble and uncertainty. The room may not always deliver, may be too full of conflicting needs to establish kindness in a consistent manner, but it will always exist; and now – here in my sixtieth year – I have a feeling of

213

urgency in needing to re-visit that mental space, before strangers move into the home my parents occupied for over fifty years of their life together.

'The way a human being's memory works,' Leopard muses, 'it's like going round in a circle?'

'In some ways – but the circle seems to get wider and wider, especially if the memories are complicated and open to interpretation. But if it's just a simple memory, like I might remember a favourite dress or pair of shoe, the circle remains the same.'

'Shoes?'

'Yes – well, I really loved pretty shoes as a child. I can describe them all in detail if you like and recall the special feeling wearing a pair of silver party shoes gave me. But that's an uncomplicated memory – it doesn't require any kind of interpretation. Each time I recall that particular pair of shoes the feeling is exactly the same.'

'Returning to your parent's house – it won't be like remembering a pair of shoes.'

'Not at all – I'm really very nervous.'

★ ★ ★

I am shaking inside with anticipation. How many years since I've been able to fully access my parent's house and garden? A sense of my father must be here – perhaps someplace upstairs, stairs I haven't climbed in years. Even the stair lift I had installed for mum is piled with clothes and old newspapers, so I've never used it.

'Are you up there dad – are you up there?'

Or maybe he's at the bottom of the garden, but the trees have grown up to the sky and the path is overgrown with weeds and brambles. I'm determined to fight through on my buggy!

'Are you out there dad – are you out there?'

This silent house is full of sound! I enter the front room which is piled high with clutter. I breathe slowly – I gather all of the ghosts together. There's quite a party going on in here! There's me aged fifteen with my friends, but my little sister is crying and hammering on the door – she feels so left out. I feel a rush of panic. She now lives the other side of the world – will have to travel thousands of miles to cross the threshold between us. I need her here – right now – we should not be clearing this home of our childhood in her absence.

The dining room smells of cigarette smoke and neglect. Every item in the room is covered with dust and grime. Cobwebs dangle, along with pieces of string that held last year's Christmas and birthday cards.

My mother's chair is eerily empty. My mind flips back in time. She is sitting there quietly crying. I have just popped in after work and dad is someplace up the garden. 'What's the matter?' I say. She looks at me with red eyes. 'I'm just sitting here thinking I've not been a very good mother.'

I am shocked. My mother is not given to guilt and rarely admits to being wrong about anything. 'Nonsense,' I say, 'of course you haven't been a bad mother.'

I have no idea if I said this to spare my mother pain or to spare myself?

'I think I'll try the stair lift,' I say to Matthew.

'Are you sure – it's a heck of a mess up there?'

My heart is pounding – a piece of my childhood and young adulthood lies up those stairs. The house seems so tiny. I now wonder how my mother coped with my moving back home with a new husband and baby when I was nineteen.

I was unwell at the time – weakened by the haemorrhaging when Stephen was just three months old.

'Ah! You didn't include that part of the story the first time round?' Leopard leaps in.

'Please try to be patient Leopard – I have no idea how this will unfold.'

I recall how we took over two rooms in the house – the front lounge and my old bedroom. Then the same again during a breakup (the first of several) when I returned home with an eighteen month old toddler and a few meagre possessions in cardboard boxes. I was heartbroken and messed up and annoyed with myself for not being able to make my relationship with Stephen's father work. My mother cared for me in a non-judgemental way.

'I'm sitting here thinking I've been a bad mother,' the ghost of my mother rattles round in my head.

'Nonsense Mum – you did your best.'

Yet I was angry with her for so long. I had craved a Kellogg's family and wanted to stay at my parents' house with Stephen and for it all to be peaceful and to have time to work my life out. But the shouting just got louder and I couldn't work anything out in the din of it all, so I had to return to my own home. The selfishness and naivety of youth; I needed my parents to be a Kellogg's family when I couldn't produce a Kellogg's family of my own!

'Perhaps *the noise* followed you – stuck to you?' Leopard suggests.

'Yes – perhaps it did. But the reasons were varied and complicated, too complicated for me to work out at the time.'

I'm nervous about entering my old bedroom. It is the bigger room at the back of the house that I first shared with my little sister, until my older sister left home. After that I inherited the small bedroom.

Every night, for a couple of years, dad had to lie on the bed with my little sister until she dropped off to sleep. This was a tense endeavour because she would kick off a hell of a storm if he tried to leave the room. My mother was tired in the evenings because there were no playgroups where a lively pre-schooler could be left for a couple of hours; no friendly social network of older mums to meet up with. It wasn't the same as living in the avenue surrounded by couples of the same age with young families. Here we were, sandwiched between Mrs Farley and another neighbour, Mr Lodge, who dad had actually 'warred' with. This was totally out of character for our father – the said incident having taken place behind a high fence between our neighbouring properties. There was a verbal altercation that resulted in Mr Lodge being laid out on the pavement. How Mr Lodge ended up supine was never clearly established.

It must have been lonely for my little sister too but she did at least have a strong will, something my older sister and I clearly lacked in our younger years as we were quite obedient.

But of course the will is still there – lies dormant.

'I hate you!' I scream at my mother one morning, slamming the door on my way out to school. I am sixteen and teenage fury has taken over from compliance. My mother is upset.

'How could she say such a thing?' she asks my father.

Two years later dad makes a fuss about driving me to the school to collect my A level results. He's agitated and grasping the steering wheel really tight and saying there's no point in any of *this* because I'm just going to get married and it will all be a waste of time. My fiancé and I sit dumbstruck in the back of the car – we have never seen my father behave uncaringly before – he has never before said an unkind word to me.

We blame my mother. My unfortunate mother is an easy receptacle for blame. She must have wound my father up over something – we figure, they must have had a row.

I am hysterical. My mother tries to calm me down. She asks if the results are alright (she can't remember what subjects I've taken). I blubber out they're good – better than I'd expected – good enough to go to university. She says, 'then that's a relief – what's the problem?'

I cry some more! The problem is I want to be fussed, for some interest to be shown, perhaps in the guise of hearty congratulations and a special cake for tea, or a card saying they are proud of me. Any little gesture really. I say I'm leaving, that college friends of my fiancé have offered me a room but three months later I'm still living at home

Things must have settled down because I don't move in with my new student friends 'till after Christmas. There's a photo of me, dad, my fiancé and my little sister sat on the settee, wearing party hats and looking happy and relaxed.

'Do you think you have a choice,' Leopard asks, 'as to what you remember?'

'Not always, but if I have the choice between focusing on a happy memory or a difficult memory I'd rather choose the happy one.'

My old bedroom doesn't look like it used to and seems to have shrunk to half its original size. A huge chest of drawers – an heirloom from my grandparents – dominates, whilst dad's single bed is piled high with clothes and other sundry items. There's another chest of drawers spewing wool and the Heath-Robinson 'fitted' wardrobes are also stuffed with our mother's wool collection.

Why do these balls of wool, in every colour imaginable, seem like hidden booty? The hoard had been the bane of dad's life – having started out in the dilapidated caravan (that my youngest sister had driven across the fields at the rear of the property and somehow lodged in the back garden). The collection multiplied and took over the pretty summer house dad erected for mum; and then in the winter months, when the balls of wool were at risk of becoming damp, it all had to be brought inside to be distributed in various cupboards throughout the house.

Bags of wool and her collection of painted pebbles – I now perceive my mother's hobbies as items of treasure. I decide the painted stones are works of art, worthy of being on display. Mum collected the pebbles from the beach during various holidays and then sat for hours meticulously painting each one with intricate symmetrical patterns. The detail is fascinating and I wonder at the patience it must have taken.

One could only achieve that level of detail in a purely meditative state. The bags of wool were no doubt destined for projects that never materialized and I think to myself that it was the colours that were the attraction.

Later – when common sense has departed and *all* the wool is stacked in *our* garden hut I find myself obsessively sorting the different shades and then I tackle the mammoth task of pairing dozens of knitting needles and placing the knitting patterns into a sense of order.

My sister buys a book on different knitting techniques and before we know it we are both clicking away knitting practice squares! Mum's interest has also been revived and she produces square after square of beautiful knitting, whilst sitting in her chair at the home. 'It's keeping my mind occupied,' she says, with a little smile. Something strange has happened since mum moved in at the care home – she's displaying an ironic wit and increased sense of humour.

We think this may be due to the fact that the home is reminding her of a familiar atmosphere she would have experienced at the hospital where she did her nurses' training. She perceives the care workers as fellow nurses and enjoys the sense of a familiar routine that mimics the caring for patients and dispensing of medication at set times. We are getting a glimpse of how our mother's personality might have been at the time dad first met her; the pretty young nurse (later awarded the Defence Medal for services to Nursing during the Second World War) who won the heart of a handsome young sergeant in the Home Guard, also a shipfitter of war ships and an excellent football player to boot.

Meanwhile, I have my own reason for knitting squares and trying to occupy my mind. Amy is very ill with a rare condition and with every stitch I'm trying to hold on to a sense of equanimity. Against this backdrop of worry we continue to try and clear mum's house.

★ ★ ★

With each visit I'm finding it hard to throw out and pass on and feel anxious that this hoarding problem is infectious – like a germ you can catch by just touching objects. Yet there's another aspect to this propensity. When our grandparents died our mother imported the entire contents of their house into her own. I'm beginning to understand this attachment to the presence of people we love in certain objects – the emotional need to hold on.

One afternoon fatigue sets in and my muscles are aching so I clear what I can from the bed in dad's room and lie down. We are discovering my mother has kept absolutely everything that ever came into her possession connected to the past; photos, postcards, memorabilia going back to her grandparents and, most important of all, the early letters between herself and our father. The letters, many of which are written in pencil on time-worn faded paper, are contained in an old red wash bag, which Matthew hands me.

'Is it all right dad?' I ask, feeling for his presence and the need to ask permission. 'Is it alright with you if I take a glimpse into those early years with mum?

Reading the letters is healing. Mum and dad had been totally in love – just as dad always told it. This was no airy, fairy romance. In the letters our parents discuss many serious issues but it is poignant to read dad's playful fantasy that when he and mum are old they will re-discover their early correspondence, in some hidden place, and read once again of their first love for each other. In a letter from later years, long after the birth of my little sister, my parents address each other in endearing words.

'I wonder what caused the tsunami?' Leopard muses.

'I'm not altogether sure Leopard – but that's probably not my story to tell.'

* * *

I rise from the bed and reach for the folding Zimmer we've bought especially for me to get round the cramped upstairs space. I have to flip one side inside itself to negotiate the bathroom. My sister has made a valiant attempt to clean the toilet area, as with the kitchen which had virtually disappeared beneath layers of dirt and clutter. Thanks to her efforts, we can at least make a cup of tea and pee in a clear space.

The small bedroom has also been tidied. It contains a single bed that dad would sometimes rest on in the afternoon and this is possibly where he occasionally wrote down his thoughts in a tattered old notebook. My sisters and I had worried about the change in pace that became apparent during the last two years of his life. When dad stopped planting seeds – the window ledges bare in the early spring months, when normally they would be covered with old margarine tubs, spouting shoots – it marked the beginnings of a downward slide.

Too few flowers and too many jumbled thoughts marked dad's demise.

★ ★ ★

Sleepy afternoon – a boiled egg and slice of toast for dinner.

'Just a little bit of dinner,' mum says, 'we don't eat much these days. No – we don't want those meals on wheels – we can manage fine.'

Sleepy afternoon – she watches Loose Women on the television and whatever follows. The voices drone on in the background – but dad isn't interested – has never bothered with the TV.

He's too tired to do the garden – sunny day outside – but his eyes feel heavy … very heavy. Stagger up the stairs – climb past the stair lift draped with clothes – shuffle across the landing piled with dresses, cardigans, trousers – everywhere clothes. His bedroom door is tied with a piece of rope – tied to mum's bedroom door. She's tied the knot tight. The cat must be on dad's bed – the cat needs his afternoon nap. Rest time – the cat on the bed, the dog in her little box – the guinea pigs scuffling in the dining room – showering sawdust on the floor – but he's too tired to clean – so very tired.

'She's kind to the guinea pigs,' he thinks, 'they sit in the palm of her hand – totally still – mesmerised – not a squeak. Will have to go in the small bedroom, can't get into my own – not allowed 'till the cat's had a sleep – the cat has to have its afternoon rest.'

Eyes heavy – feeling tired – feeling confused – he must write it all down – needs to write it down and explain … explain about the family chain – a chain is required to be strong – there mustn't be any weak links.

We must all pull together to sort out the weakest link – it has to be done. Very tired now – eyes heavy – needs to sleep.

223

'Please – can you save anything that dad's written on – even little notes on scraps of paper?' my younger sister asks over the phone. I cannot take it in that she's so far away.

'I promise,' I give her my word, and do not labour the fact that this entails going through heaps of papers and books because everything is jumbled and spread through every room in the house. I understand her request because some life force emanates in the written words and it feels hard to think in terms of throwing anything away.

This feeling even extends to letters from friends, distant relatives, people I've never met. There is a whole world being deconstructed as we clear the house – memories being torn apart from their original source.

I also remove the items my younger sister has requested from her recollections of taking over the small bedroom as a teenager. My sister has remembered a picture of Jesus surrounded by some Disney type animals that's still hung on the picture rail, a selection of cuddly toys and three dolls.

The dolls are in the bottom of the wardrobe and I realise it's the same wardrobe that stood in the small bedroom at my grandparents', the place where my grandfather stored his artificial limb. I feel a shiver run through me – just as I did as a little girl. I know if I linger ghosts will start to fill this room. Here is my older sister sat applying her mascara because the bedroom was hers before she left to be married. She dresses smartly for work as a secretary and I'm hoping the neat little sage green suit, that hangs on the same picture rail as the Disney Jesus, will get passed on to me. And here I'm sat at my desk, trying to concentrate on my school work above the distraction of raised voices, and here I am again lying in bed listening to Radio Caroline and daydreaming about who I might meet at the local disco.

I stick my head round the door of mum's bedroom. It's impossible to get in with the Zimmer and just staring at the disarray makes me feel faint. Even so, I'm expecting it to be another treasure trove. I don't sense any ghosts in this room and that feels strange. I have no memories associated with this room at all. If I'm searching for a past intimacy with my mother it lies in another house, within another time frame.

'Can we drive past the avenue,' I ask Matthew, 'just one last time?'

★ ★ ★

Leopard sighs and stretches. 'Will it be one last time?' he probes. 'This pull of memory, of nostalgia, you humans feel – it's so often laced with pain and regret.'

'Maybe we're not all grown up 'till we let go of the regret?'

'And how are you doing with that?'

'Slowly getting there – thank you.'

THIRTY TWO

2014
Our Original Face

Months pass, and as the New Year approaches, we're hoping that 2014 will prove brighter than 2013, particularly with better health for Amy.

I gather together my thoughts on what does and doesn't matter. Being there for my family and generally trying to be a caring person is high on my list. I'm acutely aware that whatever actions we make today contribute to another person's memories in the future. I particularly want to build happy connections with this house and garden for our grandchildren – just as my grandparents did for me and my sisters.

'It's easy with little children,' Leopard remarks, 'but loving grown-ups isn't always so straight forward. '

'That's true – but compassion seems to cut through a lot of the shit.'

I am still left with boxes of memorabilia from our parents' home. The paucity of childhood photographs and general family history now presents as an overflow and abundance. The room in my mind, containing happier memories and a sense of security and attachment, now opens onto many other rooms.

My son had found an envelope contained in a rusty tin box, lodged at the back of mum's wardrobe. The envelope contained our family tree on my grandmother's side. I visualise the nineteenth century parlour, the eighteenth century church where my great grand-parents married, the farm dwellings and tithed cottages of my ancestors traced all the way back to rural Northumberland in the fifteenth century.

'Don't forget us,' the voices of my ancestors cry, 'don't forget who you are and where you come from.'

There's another voice in my head, and though it may seem contradictory I don't feel that it is.

'Show me your original face – the one you had before your parents were born,' the Zen master demands in a well-known story.

Original face
As round as the moon
A circle of light
Warm like the sun
Clear
Empty
Free
No words
No pre-conceptions
No history

No baggage
Happy face
Peaceful face
Body/mind dropped off

And yet it is only a glimpse of inner freedom – this turning of the light inwards. I guess that's why meditation is called 'practice'. It's no different to building a bridge from the past to the present moment, over the turbulent waters of hurts and misunderstandings. Day by day, brick by brick, moment by moment – if we can keep our hearts open our minds can be free.

'Careful,' Leopard cautions, 'remember that promise you made me.'

'I'm sorry – just grunt, or snort, or snarl – or something, if you think I'm getting beyond myself.'

'I didn't mean to put you off, but you need to be careful with words.'

'Can I say one last thing?'

'Is it a poem?'

'Well it could be. It's just that when I look at photographs of my great grandparents, my grandparents, my parents, myself, my children and my grandchildren, I sense another aspect to this original face. There is such a strong sense of kinship and a deep pool of light in the eyes reflecting continuity through time and space and beyond.'

This deep pool of light
Within the eyes
Forget the externals,
The cheekbones

The skin
The soft hair
Framing the face.
This deep pool of light
Connecting everything
Connecting everyone
Reason enough
For being here.

THIRTY THREE

A Point of Reconciliation

The obsessive knitting of squares ceases once Amy's condition begins to improve. The wool, now sorted into myriad bags of complementary colours, is handed over to the charity shop.

The diaries are set to one side. I try to erase from my thoughts some of the unkind words written about myself, dismissing them as trivial – we all have unkind words in our minds from time to time.

My mother has reverted back to a happier time in her memories and laid her difficulties to rest, so it feels wrong to keep bitter words alive.

But I have a collection of written words I do feel the need to preserve, mainly dad's little notes, the most precious of which is written on a scrap of orange paper.

'great to see you around yesterday. I dearly love my girls and when any one of you is missing I do worry so much – I can't help it. You three are my strength. When times get rough my love, face into the winds of life dead on.'

And there are a few cards and a letter from my mother who writes, *'you're in my thoughts today and every day ...'*

I also retain the correspondence between my mother and my grandmother which astonishes me in my mother's attention to detail about our lives. It's as though we lived in our mother's head in a way that I rarely detected from her external behaviour. She writes of our achievements, our children's achievements – what they have been doing – their hopes for the future.

'Why?' I ask, 'did she not convey this interest to me?'

'Maybe you simply couldn't hear?' Leopard suggests.

'Well – I hope I can hear a little better now. It's easier because *the noise* has faded away.'

It seems we need to pick and choose fairly when thinking on the past. How would it be if the people we love remembered only our failings, could reach into our minds and drag out all of the angry, frustrated thoughts we're subject to – *all* the judgements and holier than thou sentiments – but never regarded our positive qualities?

'Hang on!' Leopard interrupts – scratching his ear. 'Erm … I just need to say – you do see the irony in what you've just said?'

'The irony involved in attempting to write a memoir that is both honest and kind? Yes, I've had quite a debate within myself concerning this. But a memoir isn't necessarily the re-telling of material facts – that wouldn't guarantee any form of honesty. The purpose of all these words isn't to emote or settle old scores, neither is it to valorise or to romanticize. If that had been the purpose this would have been a very different story – though it may still have been *my* story never-the-less.

'So what's your purpose?'

' I think just to tell a tale about milling around in the ten square feet of space that Shitou writes about in his 'Song of the Grass-Roof Hermitage'.

'But you wrote most of the story long before you found the poem?'

'I think perhaps the poem found me. I like the fact the hut ends up covered in weeds, that we can find a way to live calmly with the weeds because the weeds are the energy of life too. It just touched a nerve.'

'So you're not claiming you won't feel anger again?'

'Not at all! But later in the poem Shitou urges us to, *'Let go of hundreds of years and relax completely.'*

'Mmm … paws together and deep bows – that has to be the most calming thought I've ever considered.'

Update

These days things are calmer all round.

It's a warm day in July and Matthew is sitting at the top of the garden. He's observing the frogs in the wild life pond. In recent years our slower pace of life has allowed Matthew to become meditative. He has no religion – follows no belief system – yet his ability to 'just be' is evident.

We lead a very simple life and I occasionally feel I've done little else the past twenty-plus years other than wander up and down this small patch of a huge universe.

Sometimes – when I'm feeling confined – I imagine my buggy is a white stallion. The creature gently ambles along – pausing to look at its surroundings. It bows down to graze on sweet clover or to drink from the ponds. Then it raises its head to look at the sky, its dark eyes blinking in the rays of Sun's bright light.

My feline companion walks gracefully by the Stallion's side. Leopard's bones may be old but this takes nothing away from his sense of dignity.

'Do we always take the same walk?' I ask him.

'Of course not,' a small voice interrupts.

'She's back again,' Leopard remarks, 'but yes, I have to agree with her – it's not the same walk.'

The spirit child runs ahead. She's making a bee line for the apple tree – her favourite place of play.

'Yesterday, I saw a snail,' she calls out to us; 'it had a yellow stripe going round and round its shell. It can't be the same walk – can it, because I see something exciting and new every time?'

'Ah – the wisdom of youngsters,' Leopard murmurs, 'I wish I was a cub again.'

We all settle down at the top of the garden. It's one of those summer evenings when both Sun and Moon can be seen in the sky.

The two sisters have grown weary of their discord and wonder if the humans might one day follow suit. If the truth be told Sun and Moon long for cloud – behind the vapour screen they can rest, can dream.

'How have the humans got things so topsy-turvy?' Sun sighs. 'I mean the whole notion of *clarity* – you know – the talk of a cloudless sky, the clear light of day, and all of that? There's really nothing wrong with clouds.'

'They need the idea for song lyrics?' Moon tentatively suggests. She still doesn't quite trust Sun not to put her down. But Sun just gives a little smile of recognition before she continues.

'It's strange,' she muses, 'but there is less darkness – more light – when I close my eyes. Sometimes, I start to see ….'

For a second Sun hesitates. 'No – what I mean is – I begin to *feel* parts of the story.'

Moon shivers. 'Yes – it's hard to put into words.'

'The story,' Sun continues, 'I think it's something to do with me being you and you being me, and just everything being part of everything else.'

Moon is touched. This cosmic notion of Karma and interconnection certainly makes her irascible sister kinder! She feels sympathy for the humans who struggle with the messiness of causality, the huge responsibility the element of choice places upon them.

Leopard's ears twitch. He hears a distant sound. Sun and Moon are aware of it too.

'Can you hear the chanting?' Sun asks.

'Yes,' Moon whispers, 'it's coming from the monastery, but it doesn't belong to the monastery. I remember now – it's the bit of the story going back to the dawn of time.'

'The dawn of time and beyond,' Sun recalls.

'So this is *it*?' I say to Leopard.

'*What* is *it*?' Leopard replies.

Laughter in the apple tree.

Acknowledgements

I thank my husband Bernie for his loving support in bringing this memoir to fruition.

I also appreciate the efforts of those friends who gave the time to read and critique the manuscript, and made helpful suggestions.

The character of Leopard has been integral to my inner world for the past twenty four years so wherever Leopard is now, and may be in the future, I must also thank him and wish him safe journey.

Lightning Source UK Ltd.
Milton Keynes UK
UKOW06f0043070315

247428UK00001B/24/P